Media Programs
District and School

Media Programs
District and School

Prepared by the
AMERICAN ASSOCIATION OF SCHOOL LIBRARIANS, ALA and
ASSOCIATION FOR EDUCATIONAL COMMUNICATIONS
AND TECHNOLOGY

AMERICAN LIBRARY ASSOCIATION
CHICAGO, ILLINOIS
and
ASSOCIATION FOR EDUCATIONAL COMMUNICATIONS
AND TECHNOLOGY
WASHINGTON, D.C.

1975

This publication can be purchased from the

AMERICAN LIBRARY ASSOCIATION
50 East Huron Street, Chicago, Illinois 60611

or from the

ASSOCIATION FOR EDUCATIONAL COMMUNICATIONS
AND TECHNOLOGY
1201 Sixteenth Street, Northwest, Washington, D.C. 20036

Library of Congress Cataloging in Publication Data

American Association of School Librarians.
  Media programs: district and school.

  Includes index.
  1. Audio-visual education. I. Association for
Educational Communications and Technology. II. Title.
LB1043.A65 1975   371.33'1   74–32316
ISBN 0–8389–3159–6

Contents

Preface   vii

1   Introduction   1

2   The Media Program   4

3   Program Patterns and Relationships   10
     District Media Program   10
     School Media Program   13
     Regional Media Program   16
     State Media Program   17
     Networks   19

4   Personnel   21
     Professional Staff   22
     Support Staff   23
     District Media Staff
       and Responsibilities   25
     School Media Staff
       and Responsibilities   30
     Staffing Patterns   32

5   Operation of the Media Program   36
     Planning   36
     Budget   38
     Purchasing   42
     Production   44
     Access and Delivery Systems   48
     Maintenance   54
     Public Information   55
     Program Evaluation   58

6   Collections   62
          Selection Policies and
              Procedures   64
          Examination and Evaluation
              of Media   65

7   Facilities   87
          District Program Facilities   88
          School Program Facilities   92

8   Conclusion   105

Appendixes   109
          A   Terminology   109
          B   Acknowledgments   114

Index   123

Media Programs: District and School replaces *Standards for School Media Programs*,[1] published jointly in 1969 by the American Association of School Librarians and the Department of Audiovisual Instruction of the National Education Association (since 1971, the Association for Educational Communications and Technology). Its publication demonstrates the continuing concern of these organizations for establishing and maintaining standards of excellence in media programs in schools throughout the nation.

Both associations brought strong traditions of promoting effective guidelines for media programs to their first collaborative effort, the 1969 *Standards for School Media Programs*. This publication acknowledges further the viability of their joint effort, and through it, the Association for Educational Communications and Technology (AECT) and the American Association of School Librarians (AASL) express a mutual intent to sustain and improve school media services at every level of operation.

In the 1969 *Standards* publication, the sponsoring associations recommended that ". . . because of the rapidity of change in educational, technological, and other fields . . . national standards require continuous revision." *Media Programs: District and School* represents the response to this recommendation. Task forces were appointed by AECT and AASL in March 1971: Task Force I to revise existing standards for media programs in schools and Task Force II to develop joint standards for media programs at the district level. (*See* in Appendix B: Acknowledgments.) These documents were submitted to the boards of the two associations in the

1. American Association of School Librarians and Department of Audiovisual Instruction, National Education Association, *Standards for School Media Programs* (Chicago: American Library Assn.; Washington, D.C.: National Education Assn., 1969).

spring and summer of 1972, after which a Joint Editorial Committee was appointed to revise and edit the reports. (*See* in Appendix B: Acknowledgments.)

Recognizing the interrelationships of school and district media programs, the committee recommended that the two reports be combined into a single publication, *Media Programs: District and School*, and such action was approved by the AASL and AECT boards in their meetings in January and April 1973. Suggestions from members were obtained in open hearings conducted at the 1973 annual conferences of the associations, and the preliminary edition of the publication was circulated to members of the boards, committee chairmen, members of the two task forces, and media personnel in state departments of education.

The Joint Editorial Committee for *Media Programs: District and School*, as well as the task forces preceding it, responded as a committee of the whole to the concerns and recommendations identified by the task forces, boards, and memberships of the two associations. Most committee members belong to and are active in both AECT and AASL, further reflecting their unified efforts. Again, as in 1969, the members of the task forces and the joint Editorial Committee recommend continued periodical revision of the standards for media programs set forth here.

Media Programs: District and School reflects the thinking of many professionals in library and information science, educational technology, and related fields and represents a consensus of their perceptions of school and district media programs. Both AASL and AECT urge that media associations, persons in school media services, and other educational leaders utilize its recommendations to improve the educational opportunities of learners.

1 Introduction

The human worth that democratic societies seek to protect and develop rests upon commitment to educational programs which meet the individual purposes and developmental needs of students and prepare them to resolve the problems that continually confront them. Social, economic, and political issues, national and international, as well as the changing expectations of individuals and groups, represent the human concerns to which education must respond if it is to perpetuate and improve the society that supports it.

Those who would create better educational opportunities must strive to develop comprehensive systems that meet the needs of students of differing abilities, backgrounds, and interests, enabling them both to adjust to and influence the changing society in which they live. Media programs which reflect applications of educational technology, communication theory, and library and information science contribute at every level, offering essential processes, functions, and resources to accomplish the purposes of the school.

Media Programs: District and School delineates guidelines and recommendations for media programs and resources essential for quality education. The publication focuses on qualitative goals, offering criteria for district and school media programs that make exemplary educational experiences available to children and youth. It describes programs designed to respond to both district and school objectives and reflects the vital interrelationships between those operations. The quantitative statements that follow provide corresponding standards for the staff, collections, and facilities that are required to implement the programs. All of the recommendations apply to public and parochial school systems and to independent schools.

The guidelines are stated with recognition of alternative choices that may better serve individual program requirements. However, it should be noted that levels of program operation and the resources to maintain them were carefully analyzed, and any alternative that represents a reduction in program or in program resources is likely to result in impaired opportunities for learners.

Recommendations for the district media program identify types of resources essential for various program elements, but specific quantities are avoided since these should be determined by the size and scope of the district program. At the school level, quantitative recommendations are based on a module of 250 students and multiples thereof. Recommendations for resources to support individual school media programs are made by clustering types of resources, with a range within these clusters. On this basis, suggested staffing patterns for school media programs show alternative combinations of staff members, including media specialists, other media professionals, technicians, and aides, based on the program emphasis of individual schools. Similarly, recommendations for collections provide for ranges that reflect options available in related media formats and differing instructional emphasis. Throughout, the purpose of the guidelines is to identify media programs that are responsive to the needs and potential of effective educational programs.

Following this statement of purpose, chapter 2 defines the concept of media program and describes its essential functions. Chapter 3 discusses program patterns and relationships, considering the roles and interactions of school, district, regional, and state media programs; the role of networks and networking; and the relationship of the community to the media program. Chapters 4 through 7 present qualitative and quantitative guidelines for media program elements and resources in the form of guiding principles for each of these components and specific recommendations for their provision at the district and the individual school levels. Chapter 8 summarizes key concepts that guide the development of media programs.

Media Programs: District and School is designed to be used by media personnel and colleges and universities that prepare media professionals and teachers. It is also offered as an authoritative guide to school administrators, supervisors, business managers, boards of education, and school architects who seek responsible criteria for establishing, maintaining, and evaluating media programs. It is of value to teachers as they work with media professionals to provide the best instructional technology for learning activities. It serves students seeking to identify their role and their relationship to the human, ideological, and technological resources with which they interact. The concern for high quality education is shared by all of the people involved in the learning process and its implementation.

2 The Media Program

Programs of media services are designed to assist learners to grow in their ability to find, generate, evaluate, and apply information that helps them to function effectively as individuals and to participate fully in society. Through the use of media, a student acquires and strengthens skills in reading, observing, listening, and communicating ideas. The learner interacts with others, masters knowledges as well as skills, develops a spirit of inquiry, and achieves greater self-motivation, discipline, and capacity for self-evaluation. With a quality media program a school can challenge its members to participate in exciting and rewarding experiences that satisfy both individual and instructional purposes.

The media program exists to support and further the purposes formulated by the school or district of which it is an integral part, and its quality is judged by its effectiveness in achieving program purposes. A media program represents a combination of resources that includes people, materials, machines, facilities, and environments, as well as purposes and processes. The combination of these program components and the emphasis given to each of them derive from the needs of the specific educational program. The more purposeful and effective the mix, and the more sensitively it responds to the curriculum and the learning environment, the better the media program.

A basic component of all media programs is the human interchange among the media staff, between media staff and the administrative staff, between media staff and teachers, and most of all, between media person and student. Media personnel strive to build bridges between content and context, purpose and procedure, self and society. They apply to the achievement of learning objectives a knowledge of the potential of various information sources—verbal, symbolic, pictorial, and environmental—as well as an understanding of different teaching and learning modes. This concept of program focuses on human behaviors and interactions, with staff members supporting students and teachers and all other users in utilization of media to achieve learning goals.

Media programs contribute to the life experience of users and their individual self-fulfillment. Program evaluation requires continuous identification and appraisal of the contacts or interfacings among users and media program components, so as to determine the degree to which operational design facilitates or blocks the attainment of objectives. Effective media programs satisfy both individual and instructional purposes in a balanced and aesthetically rewarding way.

Media programs seek the widest possible uses of media resources. Within this book, the term *user*, unless otherwise limited, includes students, the professional staff, other school personnel, and as far as can be accommodated without impairing the principal goals of the program, persons in the community.

In quality media programs users are observed in all of these activities and adaptations of them:

Finding needed information on an appropriate level and in an acceptable format

Selecting and using appropriate means for retrieval of information in all media formats

Obtaining resources from the media center, district center, local agencies, and networks

Communicating in many modes, demonstrating an understanding of the structure and language of each mode

Utilizing instructional sequences of tested effectiveness to reach personal and program objectives

Designing and producing materials to achieve specific objectives, as well as using materials designed and produced for them by the media staff

Employing a variety of media to find, evaluate, use, and generate information

Enjoying the communication arts and gaining inspiration from them

Receiving assistance, both formally and informally, in the use and production of learning resources

Functioning in learning environments that reflect their developmental level as well as the tasks at hand

Locating space in which to accomplish a variety of activities responding to curricular and personal needs

Participating in the formulation and implementation of both general and specific media program policies.

The curriculum is realized and fulfilled through activities such as these. In all curriculum areas teachers and students seek information on appropriate levels and in suitable formats. They benefit from formal and informal assistance in using learning resources and designing and producing materials to achieve their objectives. Media professionals work with teachers to develop and implement curriculum design and they monitor many curricular activities of students. Increasingly, media personnel manage activities such as automated learning sequences, independent studies, graphics and film production, visual literacy programs, and seminars and other small-group activities, formerly associated largely with the classroom.

A vital concern of the media program is the guarantee of intellectual freedom for learners, teachers, and staff members. Proper preservation of human rights calls for policies and procedures that assure intellectual access to information, articulated with the approval of administrators and boards of education, and their assurance of support in carrying out these policies and procedures in ways that reflect professional integrity and skills in resolving human differences.

Activities of the media program should be considered in the light of four functions: *design, consultation, information,* and *administration.* These functions derive from the basic roles of media professionals and are overlapping rather than discrete, penetrating all operations of the program and providing a basis for evaluating their efficiency. Each of them applies to all elements of the media program but not with equal force. In describing the functions, areas of special application are identified.

The design function relates to formulating and analyzing objectives; establishing priorities; developing or identifying alternatives; selecting among alternatives; and implementing and evaluating the system, the product, the strategy, or technique. In this context media professionals initiate and participate in curriculum design. Applications of the design function are interrelated and complementary, and are viewed as cooperative action rather than the prerogative of a single staff member.

Areas calling for special consideration of the design function include:

Formulating program purposes
Establishing policies
Identifying program priorities
Generating criteria for decision-making in areas requiring judgments such as the selection of personnel, selection and circulation of materials and equipment, and technical processing
Planning and evaluating media programs
Developing the budget for the total media program
Initiating and participating in curriculum development and implementation
Designing in-service education
Developing materials for self-instructional use by learners for specified objectives
Designing multimedia presentations
Determining the effectiveness or validity of instructional materials and sequences.

The consultation function is applied as media professionals contribute to the identification of teaching and learning strategies; work with teachers and students in the evaluation, selection, and production of materials; and serve as consultants in planning and reordering physical facilities to provide effective learning environments.

Activities that are particularly affected by the consultation function are:

Participating in curriculum development and implementation
Recommending media applications to accomplish specific instructional purposes
Serving as instructional resources consultant and materials specialist

Exchanging with school personnel pertinent information regarding students' progress and problems

Developing user understanding of the strengths and limitations of various presentation forms

Planning and providing instruction in the use of the media center and its resources

Helping students develop good study habits and techniques, acquire independence in learning, and gain skill in critical thinking

Helping students develop competencies in listening, viewing, reading, and other communication skills, attitudes, and appreciations

Assisting users in the techniques of finding, using, abstracting, translating, synthesizing, and evaluating information.

The information function relates especially to providing sources and services appropriate to user needs and devising delivery systems of materials, tools, and human resources to provide for maximum access to information in all its forms.

Elements of the media program essential to the information function include:

Identifying users' needs for information

Helping users to evaluate and select materials

Organizing and indexing information

Collecting, organizing, and supplying information on community resources

Providing reference service to users

Providing bibliographic service to users

Promoting functional knowledge of the variety of resources and approaches for obtaining information

Providing access to information available from outside agencies, including networks

Providing resources and guidance in their use in response to the individual user's needs, interests, and learning styles

Translating information from one presentation form to another through production of materials.

The administration function is concerned with the ways and means by which program goals and priorities are achieved. It applies to all aspects of the program and it involves staff and users in appropriate ways.

The administration function especially serves these program activities:

Supervising media personnel
Developing media collections for school and district programs
Developing educational specifications for new facilities
Establishing access and delivery systems
Establishing and maintaining production services
Providing for maintenance of materials, equipment, and facilities
Implementing a public information program.

All media program elements reflect in varying degrees the functions of design, consultation, information, and administration. The development of an effective media program requires intelligent and perceptive application of these functions to satisfy user needs as well as provision for program operations and resources described in chapters 4 through 7.

3 Program Patterns and Relationships

Communication technology offers many choices for receiving, using, recording, and transmitting information. Full utilization of educational media makes it possible to provide alternative patterns and relationships for the instructional program that assure the "seamless curriculum" envisioned by John Dewey.

Technology presently enables the learner to participate in different environments and will increasingly do so. Television, through various distribution patterns including cable television, reaches most students in and out of school, but it is yet to serve the learning process to its full potential. Telephone lines, now used primarily for conversations or specific audience communication, have the ability to carry information into virtually every school and home. No element of the educational process needs to be limited by the walls of buildings or organizational demarcations.

Curriculum design and media utilization are inextricably interwoven. To the learner, media help to identify the problem and supply information and method to solve it. Purposeful integration of curriculum and media is ongoing and open-ended, with media professionals, curriculum consultants, teachers, and learners jointly designing instructional systems in which content and method evolve together. This process of scientific instructional design results in a more effective allocation of both the human and the material resources of the educational program.

Effective curriculum realization requires the interaction of media programs at every level—school, district, region, state—and of even farther-reaching relationships, as technology makes these possible.

District Media Program

Technological potential in a school district is best realized when the instructional applications of media and technology are placed under the administrative structure of a district media program. Such a program assumes responsibility for deployment of the total resources of instructional technology in the manner that best serves the educational goals of the district. The organizational structure places the director of the district program in a key role in decision-making related to setting overall goals, analyzing curriculum, selecting instructional modes, and establishing and maintaining responsible evaluative processes.

The responsibilities of the district media program include:

> Planning the overall media program, e.g., identifying criteria, purposes, procedures, and evaluation systems
>
> Developing and coordinating the budget for the total media program and creating and maintaining accountability techniques
>
> Applying instructional technology to curriculum development activities
>
> Selecting personnel for the district media program and providing for their ongoing professional development
>
> Orienting the district staff in all aspects of instructional technology
>
> Applying appropriate forms of telecommunications such as television, radio, telephone lines, computers, and random access distribution
>
> Developing district media selection policies that support the educational program and reflect principles of intellectual freedom
>
> Developing criteria for the selection of materials and equipment
>
> Maintaining or supervising the maintenance of media and equipment
>
> Producing materials and maintaining production facilities
>
> Selecting, distributing, and promoting effective use of district collections of materials and equipment
>
> Designing school and district media program facilities
>
> Interpreting the media program to school and community and developing public information systems.

11

In order to carry out these responsibilities, the district media program, operating as an administrative subunit, is placed in a direct line relationship to the superintendent's office. The head of the district media program may have the title of assistant superintendent, director of the district media program (the title used in this book), district coordinator of the media program, or consultant for the media program; but, regardless of designation, the person is a participating member of governing committees and councils that determine the policies and criteria for the total educational program.

All district media personnel are responsible to the director who develops staff positions and corresponding job descriptions to implement such activities as consultative services, coordination of individual school media programs, telecommunications, administration of district media collections, and district production of media. Each of these activities, to be fully developed, is headed by a media professional.

Evaluation of the district media program is the joint responsibility of the superintendent of schools and the district director, and is made on the basis of how well the program helps to set and how well it meets the educational goals of the district and individual schools. Within the program, the district director carries on further evaluation, involving the staff in identifying its operational strengths and weaknesses.

Wide variations occur in the program requirements within the district—schools serving different interests and levels of maturity, schools for children with handicaps and learning disabilities, schools for gifted children, and special purpose schools. Program elements are individually designed and evaluated on the basis of user needs and interests. The district media program seeks to accommodate and support program adaptations, encouraging the greatest possible flexibility within the parameters of effective district management. However, the district media program has the responsibility of seeing that school programs develop to their potential.

In districts where size or financial resources are insufficient for development of an adequate media program at the district level, the district should consider meeting the requirements of educational technology through such alternatives as contractual arrangements, multidistrict cooperative ventures, consolidation, or participation in

12

networks and, when possible, should seek additional funding from outside sources.

School Media Program

The school media program functions within the district media program, as well as performing as an integral part of the school's educational and administrative structure, and reflects different levels of emphasis upon specific program elements. The school program stresses direct services to students and teachers, media collections development, and instructional design that fulfills the educational goals of the school. The school media program carries out at the building level the aims of the district media program, drawing effectively on its resources. As an example, the school program conducts staff development activities, calling upon the services of district professionals as needed. Likewise, media production activities in individual schools may be complemented by more sophisticated district production services. Telecommunications activities, by nature of their function, are centered in the district program but are channeled into or coordinated with the school media program.

The school media program is conducted under the direction of a media professional, usually a media specialist with a knowledge of education and with leadership and managerial competencies, who is designated as head of the school media program. The position is placed on a direct line relationship to the principal's office. The head of a school media program has a role equal to the assistant principal or building curriculum supervisor and is a participating member of the committees and councils that determine the policies of the school.

The responsibilities of the school media program include:

Defining the purposes of the school media program with proposed implementation and evaluation to achieve them

Planning media program activities and integrating them with other programs of the school

Participating in instructional design, course development, and the creation of alternative modes of learning

13

Developing budget criteria and budget as required by the school administrator and the district media director

Developing and maintaining a balanced, relevant collection

Providing maximum access to collections in the school, district, and community

Operating the media center with procedures that further the goals of the school

Reporting to the district director, school administrator, and to teachers and students relative to the school media program

Conducting orientation and in-service education in media for the school media staff and teachers

Providing production facilities and expertise in production suitable at the school level

Developing flexible operations that encourage and support users in problem-solving, interest fulfillment, and creative expression

Initiating and providing program activities that respond to curriculum goals on a day-by-day basis

Providing opportunities for discovery and exploration independent of or beyond the stated curriculum

Maintaining professional resources for teachers, informing them about new materials, and involving them in purchasing decisions

Performing ongoing evaluations in the light of stated objectives and making program modifications as needed

Building a public relations program that communicates the role of the school media program and its contributions to the goals of the school.

A school media program, while responsible administratively to the district program, has sufficient autonomy to develop appropriate responses to differing educational requirements of the school. It seeks as its primary purpose to meet the educational goals and objectives which it has helped establish. Its program elements and staff requirements are both influenced by and contribute to the overall instructional strategies of the school. It provides curriculum designs with broad alternatives in content, method, and level of participation that require sophisticated uses of media and facilities. It recognizes and helps to establish instructional programs based on individual progress at varying rates and in different intensities that in turn may require reallocation and expansion of media resources and a larger media staff to work as members of teaching-learning teams.

The school media program occupies a unique position in helping students achieve satisfying and rewarding experiences in reading, listening, and viewing and to advance in the use of these literacies. The use and production of media provide substantial means for satisfying and expressing the personal needs and desires of students and enhancing their leisure activities. Reading competencies and growth in visual and aural literacies are essential in achieving these goals, and the media staff works with learners both independently and with teachers in helping to realize these competencies.

The school media program recognizes the need for helping learners acquire and maintain skills in researching, choosing, and using all forms of media. Media skills are the means of achieving learning goals, to be applied and practiced only in authentic learning experiences. Such skills are cumulative, and, as students progress, every media program shares the responsibility to develop and extend them.

Since the director of the district media program and the school principal share administrative responsibility for the school media program, they concur in the selection of the head of the school media program and jointly review recommendations for other media staff. In selection of media staff, the principal tends to rely on the professional judgment of the district media director and the head of the school media program.

Evaluation of the school media program is the joint responsibility of the principal, the district media director, and the head of the school media program. The principal's concern is how well the media program responds to the total program of the school and specifically meets the needs and satisfies the interests of its users. The district director seeks to measure the response of the school program to district goals and objectives. The head of the school media program ascertains the quality of the program, its fulfillment, and how effectively it amalgamates school and district media program goals.

Regional Media Program

During the past decade a rapid growth of regional media programs has taken place, some conducted as subunits of regional organizations offering broad educational services, others concerned solely with media and technological services. Regional media programs have developed under varying auspices and reflect differences in administrative structures and relationships to district media programs. A regional media program may function as an intermediate agency of a state department of education media program; it may derive from state legislation but be a virtually autonomous operation; or it may develop from cooperative efforts of local school districts, supported by combinations of local, state, and federal funds.

Regardless of its organizational pattern, the regional media program exists to provide services which school districts cannot provide for themselves or to strengthen school district programs by supplementing existing services or offering superior alternatives. For some districts the regional media center serves as a substitute for the district media program; for others it is supplemental; and a number of districts may have little or no need for regional services.

Although regional media programs differ, they generally offer many services similar to those provided by district media programs. These responsibilities may be assumed by a regional program:

Providing advisory, consultative, and informational services

Technical processing

Building special collections and providing duplicate copies for high-use situations

Providing comprehensive or selective examination collections of instructional materials, purchased and/or obtained on loan for the use of their clientele

Producing educational radio and television programs

Serving as centers for computerized instruction, remote access distribution systems, mobile units, and the like

Carrying out staff development programs for media professionals and teachers.

To ensure that regional media programs reinforce district and school program goals and respond to the needs of the region, representatives of all user groups participate actively in establishing policies for governing and financing the regional program. Some regional programs are particularly vulnerable to temporary fluctuations in funding and in funding sources; this limits their effectiveness and should be remedied wherever possible. Participating school districts should be prepared to assure the continuance of regional media programs that are providing valuable services responsive to user needs. The district media program has the responsibility of negotiating arrangements with regional media programs.

A regional media program functions in harmony with the media program of the educational agency of the state in which it operates.

State Media Program

The state is legally responsible for establishing and maintaining a system of education and the education agency prescribed by its legislature to provide leadership in the area of media programs. Extensive variations exist among the states in number and size of schools and school districts and types of organization, and their goals and purposes are further influenced by geographic conditions, socioeconomic factors, and potential resources. The result is a wide variance in the development of media programs, but in all instances these programs are the responsibility of the state educational agency.

The state board of education generates creative policies for media programs and is responsible for making recommendations for legislative action that insures the provision of resources necessary for media program development. Such policies are implemented in the state department of education by an adequate media staff functioning as a unit which encompasses the total resources of educational technology, including instructional telecommunications. The administrative subunit for the state media program is placed in a direct line relationship to the office of chief state school officer. The administrator of the state media program is a participating member of committees or councils charged with departmental and educational planning.

17

The Council of Chief State School Officers[1] exhibits continuing leadership in motivating state departments of education to expand and improve their roles in the media field. The council identifies as primary responsibilities of the media program in the state department of education the interpretation and implementation of policies of the state board of education and state and federal laws and regulations relating to media in the educational program including:

Planning for effective media programs

Developing standards for media programs

Making budget recommendations based upon needs assessment

Developing guidelines for administration of federal and state funds

Providing consultative services for program and staff development for the state department of education, school districts, professional associations, and lay groups interested in education

Organizing and encouraging leadership development programs

Establishing criteria to assist local school districts in evaluating media

Producing instructional materials not available from other sources

Planning state television programs and networks

Evaluating media programs

Collecting, analyzing, and disseminating information to the chief state school officer, the state board of education, state department of education staff, state legislators, congressmen, local school districts, and the general public

Planning and developing research programs relating to media

Coordinating media activities with other units of the state department of education, such as research, curriculum, and school planning units

1. Council of Chief State School Officers (CCSSO), *Developing the Use of New Educational Media* (Washington, D.C., The Council, 1964).

> Participating in the development of certification require-
> ments for media personnel
>
> Assisting with planning for media education in colleges
> and universities
>
> Working with state and national groups such as pro-
> fessional associations, public libraries, state library
> agencies, networks, and the U.S. Office of Education.

The media program in the state department of education seeks to promote exemplary professional practices in regional, district, and school programs. School districts call upon the services of the state media unit to strengthen their development at the district and school levels; likewise, state media units exert leadership in establishing and maintaining media programs in their best and most efficient forms in regional, district, and school programs.

Networks

A network is a system for providing access to data bases. Its purpose is to increase users' access to information and information sources. A data base is developed by identifying the location and availability of information in participating agencies which may include schools, school districts, colleges and universities, public libraries and regional library systems, and state, national, and international agencies. Networks transcend geographic or political divisions or subdivisions and may be local, regional, statewide, national, or international in scope.

A media program at the district or school level may be affiliated with a network either by contracting for services as needed or by membership subscription. As networks develop, media programs of school districts participate actively in policy decisions on the nature and origin of information sources and services to be offered by the network. The director of the district media program is responsible for maintaining liaison with networking agencies and calls upon the school district to supply adequate funding for network participation.

The network furnishes access to information or knowledge not readily available to regional, district, and school programs. This information, usually in verbal form, may be transmitted by advanced communication techniques such as telecommunications, computer systems, or high-speed random access retrieval systems. The Educational Resources Information Center (ERIC) which disseminates information about educational research projects, research-related materials, and other educational resource information, and the Machine-Readable Cataloging (MARC) program of the Library of Congress are examples of national networks.

The media centers of systems of special education and other systems for interlibrary loan are examples of networks established to provide information on the location and availability of particular resources useful in instructional programs.

4 Personnel

Realization of the purposes of the media program depends on the quality and extent of the personnel who are employed to implement the media program. Personal and professional competencies are basic ingredients of every media-oriented operation.

GUIDING PRINCIPLES

1. Media staff at both district and school levels are in the vanguard of educational programs and practices, participating in and encouraging innovative teaching and learning practices.
2. Media professionals, as members of the instructional staff, make instructional decisions within their purview and provide appropriate leadership in the educational process.
3. Differentiated staffing that provides a full range of professional, technical, and clerical competencies is necessary to implement a media program.
4. Staff in sufficient number is an indispensable part of a functional media program.
5. Every school district employs at the district level at least one full-time media professional who provides leadership for the development of the media program.
6. Every school employs at least one full-time media specialist who serves as head of the school media program.
7. Media staff has status, salary, fringe benefits, and working conditions equal to that of other staff members with comparable qualifications and responsibilities.

TYPES OF PERSONNEL

Personnel for creating and maintaining educational media programs include the professional staff and the support staff.

Professional Staff

All media personnel who qualify as *professional*, whether certificated or not, are included in this category. The word *professional* identifies abilities, skills, and knowledges including appropriate academic preparation, a disposition to problem solving, expertise in one or more areas of educational technology or library and information science, personal efficiency, effective human relationships, and participation in professional associations. The term *media professional*, as used in this book, therefore includes all persons whose attributes, training, and experience render them professional.

MEDIA SPECIALIST

A media specialist has broad professional preparation in education and media, has appropriate certification, and possesses the competencies to initiate and implement a media program. The media specialist holds a master's degree in media from a program that combines library and information science, educational communications and technology, and curriculum. This academic preparation develops competencies relating to:

> The role of education in society
> Theories, principles, and methods of instructional technology
> Curriculum development and teaching and learning strategies
> Analysis of user characteristics and information needs
> Principles of communication
> Principles for disseminating and using information
> Planning and administering media programs
> Materials and information services for children and young adults, including reference and bibliography
> Content analysis and oral interpretation of materials

Techniques for guiding users in reading, listening, and
viewing
Organization of information, i.e., cataloging and classi-
fication
Information processing, storage, and retrieval systems
Media design and production
Interpretation and application of research.

OTHER MEDIA PROFESSIONALS

A person also qualifies as a media professional when he or she has
had academic preparation and experience in an area of educational
technology or information science, such as instructional development, instructional television, computer technology, media production, programmed instruction, and technical processes. While not
all media professionals need to be certificated by the state, their
programs of preparation must include curriculum and instruction
(and other appropriate areas of professional education) as well as
their media specialities. Certainly, media professionals with career
objectives of head of a school media program or director of a district media program must have a broad preparation and background
in education in addition to media expertise. Although the intent of
Media Programs is to encourage leadership potential in all media
professionals, certification requirements should insure selection of
heads and directors of programs who have appropriate educational
backgrounds and experience.

Support Staff

The support staff of the media program consists of technicians
and media aides. They are responsible to the media professionals,
but occupy identified positions with job descriptions that delineate
their duties. The support staff provides essential services that require
a general knowledge of media program functions as well as specific
skills necessary for the performance of duties. Preparation for the
position of technician or media aide is acquired either by specialized
training or on-the-job experience.

MEDIA TECHNICIAN

Media programs require personnel with a variety of technical qualifications, training, and experience in particular fields. Technicians have competencies in one or more fields such as graphics production and display, information and materials processing, photographic production, operation and maintenance of instructional equipment, television production, and installation of system components. Typical duties of media technicians include:

> Assisting in the technical processing of information and materials by performing such tasks as bibliographic searching and processing of materials
>
> Producing graphics and display materials such as transparencies, posters, charts, graphs, displays, exhibits, and materials for television programs
>
> Performing photographic production work such as still photography, motion photography for films and television, developing black-and-white film
>
> Installing system components such as closed-circuit television systems and film chains
>
> Repairing and maintaining equipment
>
> Providing instruction in the operation and use of instructional equipment.

MEDIA AIDE

Aides have secretarial and clerical competencies that enable them to perform tasks related to the ordering, receipt, maintenance, inventory, production, circulation, and utilization of materials and equipment. Media aides working directly with users must be able to respond effectively to their needs. They carry out all tasks under the direction of the professional members of the media staff, reporting, as appropriate, to designated professionals or technicians. Typical duties of media aides include:

> Preparing, processing, and receiving orders
>
> Processing materials
>
> Maintaining records, inventories, and bookkeeping accounts

Typing correspondence, reports, and bibliographies

Locating and retrieving materials and equipment for users and assisting them in using media center resources

Assisting in the production of materials, e.g., transparencies, models, audiotapes

Assisting in the operation and minor repair of equipment and in the maintenance and repair of materials

Shelving, filing, and duplicating materials

Checking lists and bibliographies to determine availability of materials

Performing circulation tasks such as charging, discharging, reserving, booking, scheduling, and delivery of materials and equipment

Responding to the needs and interests of students under the supervision of the head of the media center.

As a media program expands, the need increases for technicians and aides with specialized preparation in such areas as information and materials processing, graphics design and production, reprographic techniques and displays, photography and other media production methods, television production (including videotaping and studio production), electronics, and computerized operations.

District Media Staff and Responsibilities

The size of the district and the scope of its program determine the number and range of media staff positions. The staff reflects the professional, technical, and clerical competencies required to implement all of the program elements.

The staff works under the direction of the district media director with participatory management practiced by delegating authority and responsibility to subordinate levels where decisions can be made effectively and with proper accountability. The management system insures participation by clear delineation of positions and lines of communication and responsibilities.

Cooperation among school districts influences staffing needs. It is unrealistic for every school district to attempt to provide by itself the full range of media-program elements needed for teaching and learning. Possibilities for mutually advantageous contractual arrangements between school districts should be explored, as, for example, a group of school districts setting up a cooperative technical processing center to handle purchasing, cataloging, and processing of materials for all of their schools. One or more districts may develop extensive film collections available to all schools within a multi-district area. Regional curriculum laboratories and educational media selection centers may be provided. Regional and state telecommunications systems can be developed. The use of any of these alternative patterns modifies staffing needs at the district level.

DISTRICT MEDIA DIRECTOR

The district media director is a media professional chosen on the basis of breadth of knowledge and experience in media programs; managerial, administrative, and supervisory competencies; and concern for the fulfillment of the purposes of education. This person occupies the key position in bringing to the educational program the full application of media and technology.

The responsibilities of the director of the district media program are varied and complex. The director

> Provides leadership in all aspects of the district media program and delegates responsibilities to appropriate personnel
>
> Is a participating member of the superintendent's governing committees or councils for curriculum and instructional planning
>
> Plans or coordinates the planning of an effective media program, based on analysis of the goals and objectives of the district's instructional program
>
> Acts as the leader for the heads of school media programs, providing at the district level examples of the professional support that those persons must in turn supply for their staff and users at the school level, including recognition, idea exchange, counselling, and expectation of achievement of objectives
>
> Coordinates the district media program with the total educational program and with other information services at community and higher levels

Determines priorities for the total media program (district and school levels)

Develops and administers the budget for the total media program

Establishes position classifications for media personnel at the district and school levels

Receives recommendations for staff appointments and selects or participates in selection and evaluation of personnel

Provides staff development opportunities for media staff and other school personnel at district and school levels

Coordinates planning for media program facilities

Designs and implements a public information program

Plans and coordinates ongoing evaluation of the media program.

DISTRICT STAFFING PATTERNS

Because of the many variables within school districts, a specific organization of operations and staff components is not presented here. In small districts some operations and staff responsibilities are combined and/or provided on a contractual basis with other districts or agencies. Large districts maintain more extensive operations, but may also find it advantageous to provide some program elements through contractual arrangements or utilization of regional or state-level services. Typical district media operations and staff needs are outlined forthwith.

PLANNING AND ADMINISTRATION. District media program activities are directed by a media professional who provides leadership for the development of district-level and individual school media programs. Additional professional media personnel are employed as needed to administer specific program operations. The professional staff is supported by sufficient secretarial staff.

CONSULTATIVE SERVICE AND STAFF DEVELOPMENT. Competent advice and assistance in the development and utilization of media programs is provided to the heads of school media programs and other school personnel, including members of the district staff, school administrators, media personnel, and teachers. Staff development programs are conducted for media staff and other school personnel.

27

FILM, VIDEOTAPE, AND RELATED COLLECTIONS. Collections of 16mm films, videotapes, and other materials for loan to individual schools are administered under the direction of a media professional assisted by support staff (booking clerks, film inspectors, distribution clerks) as needed. The staff is adequate in number and variety of competencies to insure that users have convenient and timely access to titles in the collection and that no more than twenty-four hours is required for the return, inspection, and redistribution of materials. Factors influencing the size of staff include the number of schools/teachers/students served, geographic characteristics of the district, size of the collection, booking procedures, and technology used.

PROFESSIONAL LIBRARY. The professional library for the district is administered by a media specialist assisted by additional professional staff and media aides. The number of users, the scope and depth of services provided, such as handling telephone requests and performing research and abstracting services, and provisions for extended hours of operation determine the number of persons that are needed.

MEDIA SELECTION AND EVALUATION CENTER. The district media selection and evaluation center is administered by a media specialist assisted by media aides and, in larger operations, by staff with professional competencies in specific subject areas. This center may be operated in conjunction with the district professional library or may form a separate subunit of the district media program.

PROCESSING CENTER. A district processing center is administered by a professional in technical processing of information and materials with managerial competencies. The staff includes catalogers, media technicians (library technical assistants), and media aides as needed. The number of new titles cataloged, the number and types (formats) of materials cataloged and processed, data processing techniques and equipment employed, and the depth of cataloging and processing provided are conditions that affect the size and quality of staff. Alternatives include the use of commercial cataloging and processing services or contracting with other districts or agencies for processing services.

EQUIPMENT SERVICES. Equipment services provided at the district level include evaluating and maintaining equipment, distributing specialized equipment on loan to individual schools, and lending temporary equipment to cover for items being serviced or repaired. The equipment program is administered by a media professional; additional professional staff may be required for equipment evaluation. Media technicians perform equipment maintenance, unless it is provided through contractual arrangements with commercial agencies.

MEDIA PRODUCTION. Media production operations at the district level may include graphics, printing, photography, television and radio, and audiotape production services. These operations interrelate in terms of staff competencies. They are outlined separately to identify staffing requirements (but not to prescribe organizational patterns).

> *Graphics*: The district media program provides graphics production services giving leadership to and also supplementing production activity at the individual school level. Graphics production is administered by a media professional. Supporting staff includes graphics artists, other technicians, and aides, and the number needed is influenced by how many teachers and other school personnel are served, as well as the scope of production services.
>
> *Printing*: When printing services needed by the school district relate to the instructional program in the preparation and production of instructional material, consideration should be given to incorporating printing services within the district media program. The decision is influenced by the instructional needs to be served by printing, existing practice and its adequacy, the volume and complexity of printing required, and the degree to which needed equipment, processes, and staff competencies overlap those required for other media production activities. Staff for fully developed printing services includes a manager, editors as needed, qualified operators for photography, printing, and binding, and typesetters for any typesetting units employed. Alternatives include the services of a commercial company or a technical school that teaches printing skills, or the provision of printing

services by a district unit separate from the media program.

Photography: District photography services to supplement photography performed at the individual school level are administered by a media professional. The supporting staff includes photographers, graphics artists, other technicians, and aides as needed.

Television and radio: District television services, including assistance to school personnel in television utilization, are administered by a media professional. The types and size of staff for district television services are determined by such factors as methods employed for use of television, the extent of television program production at the district level (as compared to use of programs produced at regional or other levels, and production within individual schools), the degree of assistance needed in individual schools, and the extent to which noncommercial television programs are taped for later use. Extensive districtwide television production, either broadcast or closed-circuit, requires employment of engineers, technicians, clerical staff, television teachers, script writers (employed for specific productions), and graphics production support staff as needed. Apprentice production crew members, such as students enrolled in community college or vocational-technical courses in television and radio, can be employed for support positions, when appropriate. Alternatives to consider include use of programming from regional, state, and other sources, as well as contracting for specific television productions.

Audiotape production: Audiotape production and duplication services are administered by a qualified media professional, with technicians and aides as needed.

School Media Staff and Responsibilities

The size of the school and the scope of its program determine the extent of the school media program staff. It reflects school organization such as the open school, departmental management in high schools, specialized services, and programs to accommodate and mediate learning disabilities and physical handicaps. It also is affected by the allocation of program activities and services between the district and the individual schools.

RESPONSIBILITIES OF THE HEAD OF THE SCHOOL MEDIA PROGRAM

The head of the school media program is a media specialist selected on the basis of managerial and administrative competencies, coupled with a wide knowledge of media and expertise in instructional design. This person is responsible for developing, administering, and implementing a full media program. In large schools with a varied professional media staff, the head of the program may be a media professional other than a media specialist. In such cases, selection of the program head is based on the person's breadth of knowledge, experience, and leadership capabilities.

The head of the school media program

Plans and administers the school media program, working cooperatively with the principal, the district media director, other media staff, and users, delegating duties and appropriate authority to members of the school media staff

Reports to the school administrator and works with administrative staff in planning ways to improve instruction

Sustains lines of communication established by the district media director and consults freely with that office

Plans and implements media program policies

Works with the district media director to coordinate the school media program with other school media centers, libraries, and agencies in the community

Participates in the school's governing committee or council for curriculum and instructional planning

Works as a member of curriculum committees, textbook committees, and other instructional groups

31

Develops, proposes, and justifies budget requests for the school media program, in consultation with media staff members, principal, and district media personnel

Assists with the selection of personnel for the school media program

Provides media staff development programs and evaluates staff performance

Provides staff development programs for teachers in the evaluation, selection, and use of materials

Serves as chairman of the media center advisory committee(s)

Coordinates the formulation of the school's media selection policy in accordance with district policy

Coordinates the selection, organization, and distribution of materials and equipment

Develops a climate that encourages students and teachers to take full advantage of the media center and its resources

Interprets the school media program to students, faculty, administration, and community.

Staffing Patterns

Because of differences in school size and the scope and depth of media programs, a specific organization of the school media staff is not presented here, but basic program requirements call for professional personnel, technicians, and aides. The school media staff must be competent to work with users with differing interests and needs; to respond to a wide span of instructional approaches; and to manage a variety of resources. When a single media specialist supported only by technicians and aides carries on the total media program of a school, that person must have a wide spread of competencies and professional skills. School media programs employing two or more media professionals profit from selecting individuals who have complementary specializations, thereby increasing the capabilities of the program.

Employment of sufficient technical and clerical staff to work under the guidance of media professionals is essential to program realization and to promote efficient and economical staffing. Technicians and aides perform a variety of essential, time-consuming tasks, contribute to the efficient operation of the media program, and release professionals to work in the areas of their expertise.

Patterns of organization for instruction and systems of instructional technology influence the allocation of media staff responsibilities. Alternative approaches include assignment of staff to work with specified grade-level, age-level, or multiaged groups; with subject area specializations; with special subschool organizations; or with specific blocks of instruction.

The program of a large school may be extended by subject resource centers developed as satellites to the main media center. Each resource center requires a media specialist with appropriate subject matter competencies. This person is responsible to the head of the school media program who provides support staff as needed and oversees and coordinates the program of satellite centers with the total school media program.

SIZE OF STAFF

Recommendations for size of staff for the school media program are influenced primarily by the number of users—students, teachers, and others—served by the school media program. Other variables that influence media staff needs include instructional approaches and emphasis; patterns of school organization; provisions for resource centers as satellites to the main media center; media program operations in such areas as television production and materials design and production; services provided by the district media program; and the level of use of the media program and its resources.

The professional staff, consisting of the head of the school media program and other media personnel as needed, is sufficient in number and variety of competencies to insure that the media program is planned carefully and implemented fully; that resources for teaching and learning are selected wisely and are made easily accessible; and that individualized media services to students and teachers are provided in optimum measure.

Each school with an enrollment of 250 students requires a full-time media specialist. Additional professional staff members are required to respond to the needs of users in schools with larger en-

33

rollments and to provide a full range of media services. One full-time media professional for every 250 students (or major fraction thereof) can implement a fully developed media program. This figure is recommended rather than prescribed, but it should be noted that it is based on analysis of tasks to be performed and the time required to perform them.

Personnel requirements vary with circumstance. Schools with enrollments exceeding 2,000 students may find it possible to achieve a full complement of professional competencies and satisfy user needs with less than one professional for every 250 students. In other schools, the number of media specialists and other media professionals may have to be increased because of such factors as a student body with special learning problems, provisions for satellite resource centers, and emphasis on such media production services as graphics, radio, and television. Very small schools with one and two teachers in sparsely populated areas present unique problems in staffing for which the school district needs to devise alternatives to the full-time staffing pattern.

New schools require media programs comparable to those recommended for established schools. To have the media center in full operation when the new school opens requires advance planning with sufficient time and funds provided for this purpose. Appoint-

TABLE 1.   RECOMMENDED STAFFING PATTERNS

SCHOOL ENROLLMENT	PROFESSIONAL STAFF		
	HEAD OF MEDIA PROGRAM	ADDITIONAL MEDIA PROFES- SIONALS	SUBTOTAL
250	1	0	1
500	1	0–1	1–2
1,000	1	2–3	3–4
1,500	1	3–5	4–6
2,000	1	4–7	5–8

(a) The balance of media professionals with specialized competencies to technicians depends somewhat on the quality of the support staff.

ment of a full-time media specialist and media aide to work a year in advance of the opening of a new school is essential for providing an operational media program.

Support staff of media technicians and media aides should be sufficient in size and in variety of competencies to insure that the media program operates efficiently, that sufficient technical and clerical skills required to perform particular media services are available, and that the time of media professionals is not usurped to perform support-level tasks.

Each school with an enrollment of 250 needs a full-time media aide and, in most cases, a full-time media technician. A ratio of two full-time support staff members for every 250 students (or major fraction thereof) is recommended to fully implement a well-developed media program, again based on analysis of the tasks to be performed and the time required to perform them.

Adjustments in levels of support staffing or the ratio of aides to technicians depend on the needs of particular schools. The number of media technicians may be increased because of extensive media production services and the number of aides increased to accommodate provisions for satellite resource centers.

Table 1 illustrates options in staffing school media programs to respond to user needs.

FOR SCHOOL MEDIA PROGRAMS

	SUPPORT STAFF		TOTAL STAFF
MEDIA TECHNICIANS (a) (b)	MEDIA AIDES	SUBTOTAL	
1	1	2	3
1–2	2–3	3–4	4–6
3–5	3–5	6–8	0–12
4–6	4–6	8–12	12–18
5–8	5–8	10–16	15–24

(b) The number of media technicians is influenced by the services provided from the district media program and by program emphasis within the school.

35

5 Operation of the Media Program

This chapter presents guidelines and recommendations for district media program and school media program operations, including *planning, budget, purchasing, production, access and delivery systems, maintenance, public information,* and *program evaluation.* Each section proceeds from statements of guiding principles to specific qualitative and quantitative recommendations for the district and school program.

Interrelationships between district and school, as well as region, state, and other levels, are reflected in the qualitative and quantitative recommendations. As an example, when staff development is centered at the district level, lesser emphasis is needed in individual schools. Or, where extensive provision for electronic maintenance service exists at the district level it reduces the individual schools' need for media technicians to perform maintenance and repair. Similarly, the scope of district technical services for cataloging and processing materials influences the number of building media technicians and aides required for this activity.

The autonomy of the school media program and the importance of its ability to serve its community is always recognized in other operations such as collections development and program activities that fulfill individual student needs, course goals, and the overall purposes of the school. Such operations are influenced to a lesser degree by the district program but the school program has its full support in achieving them.

Planning

Planning for media programs is a cooperative effort of district and school media professionals working with other professional members of the educational staff and the users of media resources. It pervades every operation of program development rather than constituting a single step or stage.

GUIDING PRINCIPLES

1. The media program reflects, supports, and also helps to determine the goals and objectives of the educational program of which it is an integral part.
2. Planning for the media program is based on users' needs and interests.
3. Planning for the media program sets priorities within its delineated program objectives.
4. Decisions leading to ways to respond to identified needs are based on systematic analysis of alternatives, constraints, and other variables.
5. Planning is a cooperative process involving media program administrators, media staffs, school administrators, teachers, students, and community members, as appropriate.
6. Planning is continuous and iterative and is the means through which program elements are selected, implemented, and evaluated in relation to program objectives, which are also being continuously reviewed.
7. The planning process guides all aspects and stages of media program development from formulation of goals through evaluation of the effectiveness of specific program components and operations.

Development of effective media programs at district and school levels requires an understanding of user needs and interests and instructional design, a clear definition of program goals and objectives, and a knowledge of available and needed resources. Systematic planning establishes both short- and long-range goals of the media program as well as the means and measures for achieving its objectives.

An analysis of user needs and interests provides a sound data base for decision-making relative to setting goals, modifying them, and devising program strategies. When this assessment is ongoing it avoids unwarranted expenditures of resources on short-lived demands. Activities and resources that constrain effective programming are replaced with appropriate alternatives. A continuous planning cycle includes total program evaluation and results in the validation, modification, and/or replacement of elements as needed.

The director of the district media program is responsible for the overall design of the media programs of the district and for assuring appropriate participation and cooperation in the design process. District planning provides for diversity in programming and alternative solutions to educational problems, encouraging schools to respond to the unique characteristics of their particular community.

The head of the school media program is similarly responsible for planning the school media program, and for assuring appropriate participation and cooperation in the design process. The school program head works in close cooperation with the media staff, principal, and all users. School-level planning is designed to meet the needs of a specific population; it also reflects the overall goals of the district media program. Thus the head of the school media program brings together inputs from the school and the district media program and creates a program that reflects in a compatible way both sets of goals.

District media program planning and school media program planning build into their design methods of measuring how effectively the programs achieve their declared objectives. Every media program responds to accountability procedures created by the administrations to which it reports, but media professionals also recognize an internal obligation to the principle of accountability in designing plans that require them to measure their own program achievements.

All areas of media program operations, considered in more detail in the sections which follow, are shaped by the planning process.

Budget

Budgeting is the financial aspect of planning for the media program. The budget identifies specific program objectives based on user needs, identifies resources required to accomplish these objectives, and presents the financial requirements for supplying these resources.

GUIDING PRINCIPLES

1. The media program is an integral part of the instructional program rather than a support service and the media budget provides the resources for teaching and learning.
2. The director of the district media program is responsible, within established administrative channels, for the design, formulation, justification, administration, and evaluation of the budget for the media program in the district.
3. The head of the building media program works with the principal in creating budget recommendations to submit to the district director.
4. The media program budget is developed cooperatively and is based on program goals and objectives.
5. Budget preparation applies systems theories that emphasize program and accountability.
6. The total media program budget includes funds for both school and district programs, with fiscal responsibility assigned at the appropriate operating level.
7. Where decentralization places budgeting for media program resources under the individual school, the head of the school media program, the principal, and the district media director concur in its approval.
8. The responsibility for identifying or approving funding sources, including state, federal, and local funds, rests at the district level.
9. Implementation of the budget is carried out in accordance with local, state, and federal laws and regulations governing purchases, contracts, bidding procedures, building codes, and standards of operations.

Media program budgets are developed primarily by media professionals, but they work with other professional personnel and consider the suggestions and needs of teachers, students, administrators, consultants, and citizen groups. The media staff considers various theories of budgeting and reconciles with the business office a system that properly reflects the goals and objectives of the planning process. Planning–programming–budgeting system (PPBS), performance budgeting, and cost-effectiveness analysis are examples of systems with applications to budgeting for the media program.

The budget presentation emphasizes the relationship of resources to program capabilities leading to desired learner outcomes. To support requests, explanations and justifications are included and expressed, when possible, in terms of learning objectives, i.e., as learner outputs rather than resource inputs. In school districts that employ a traditional function-object (line item) format for budgets, the media program budget may be prepared in dual form, using a program budget to accompany the traditional budget, thereby demonstrating the relationship of line item requests to specified objectives of the educational program.

Budget allocations include the funds needed to support operations, the district media program, individual school media programs, and any regional program or network to which the district may subscribe. They also include operating funds for ongoing program support and capital outlay funds for major initial expenditures such as construction and remodeling of media center facilities, acquisition of initial collections of materials, and equipment for new schools. Ongoing program allocations provide support for personnel, materials, equipment, supplies, facilities, maintenance, contractual arrangements, and other resources as needed. If district organizations and regulations cause individual schools to budget for some of these items, the district media program director works with the principal and the head of the school media program to develop adequate media program funding.

The director of the district media program and the head of the school media program should investigate alternative possibilities for funding within and outside the district, including the use of state, federal, and local funds. A proposal for funds for an individual school should be jointly approved by the district media program director, the school administrator, and the head of the school media program.

To maintain an up-to-date collection of materials and equipment that fulfills and implements the instructional program, the annual per student expenditure of a school district should be at least 10 percent of the national Per Pupil Operational Cost (PPOC), as computed by the United States Office of Education. According to the USOE definition, the PPOC includes the cost of administration, instruction, attendance services, health services, pupil transportation services, operation of plant, maintenance of plant, and fixed charges, computed on average daily attendance.

The standard of 10 percent of the PPOC for annual expenditures for materials and equipment is expressed as a single figure, based on recommendations from school administrators, school business managers, and media professionals. It reflects the essential relationship between materials and the equipment required for their use, and it provides the flexibility needed to achieve balanced collections and to respond to the differing needs of individual schools and districts. All allocated funds are expended for the district program and individual school programs on the basis of program needs.

This standard for annual expenditures for collections provides for the acquisition of newly published or produced materials, needed materials other than those currently released, replacements of titles, duplicates, media production supplies, the costs for preprocessing of materials, and items of equipment (e.g., projectors, viewers, radio and television receivers, microform readers, record players, audio-tape recorders, screens, projection stands, media production equipment, and the like). For budget purposes, the line labeled *collection* includes all materials, equipment, and operational supplies. This figure *does not include* funds needed for such items as installation of expensive electronic facilities, general school supplies, delivery systems, security and insurance costs, plant and equipment maintenance, initial collections for new schools, school-adopted textbooks purchased for each student, salaries of media staff, public information programs, furniture, and special laboratory equipment.

Funds for initial collections of materials and equipment in newly established media centers are provided from capital outlay, rather than from the amount recommended for annual per pupil expenditures for collections. Schools in which media center collections do not meet current standards for size and quality require additional funds to augment the annual budget until adequate collections have been built.

The recommendation for annual expenditures takes into consideration materials and equipment needed to implement school programs which stress individualization, independent study, and inquiry.

41

Additional funds may be needed to meet the requirements of special programs and curricular experimentation.

Districts and schools whose operating costs are less than the national Per Pupil Operation Cost figure should consider an appropriation for collections based on the larger amount so that it provides adequate resources for teaching and learning. Districts and schools spending more than the national figure should use their own per pupil operating cost as the base for the 10 percent appropriation for collections so as to maintain collections capable of supporting a superior instructional program.

Purchasing

Purchasing encompasses the entire operation of supplying the nonhuman resources of the total media program. It calls for business acumen coupled with a knowledge of materials and equipment and a sensitivity to the overall program goals as reflected in the budget.

GUIDING PRINCIPLES

1. Purchasing for district and school media programs is coordinated by the director of the district media program acting upon recommendations and requests from the heads of the school media programs.
2. Centralized purchasing is used wherever it best serves the goals of the total educational program.
3. Purchasing policies and procedures recognize the essentiality of the head of the school media program being able to respond to the instructional design and program goals of the school.
4. Purchasing policies and procedures provide for acquisition of materials, equipment, and supplies at the time of need, including items required on short notice.
5. Purchasing policies encourage rather than restrict convenience in purchasing inexpensive consumable items at both school and district levels.
6. Purchasing policies and procedures provide for evaluation of materials and equipment prior to purchase.

7. Purchasing policies and procedures provide needed items at the best available price consonant with efficient and effective service from the supplier.
8. The district media program director knows and applies existing state laws and regulations and district policies and procedures relating to purchasing.

The director of the district media program, working through appropriate administrative channels, coordinates the acquisition of materials, equipment, and supplies for the total media program, including items selected by the individual schools and those selected for the district program. In this process the director both involves and is involved with the heads of school media programs in acquiring input on specialized needs, applications of media and equipment, and the performance and effectiveness of purchases.

MATERIALS. Purchasing practices provide needed materials, without substitution of titles, at the best available price compatible with efficient and effective service from the supplier. Purchase of materials from jobbers usually results in significant savings. The bid procedure is not recommended for the supply of books and related materials.[1]

EQUIPMENT AND SUPPLIES. In districts where a bid procedure is required by state law or district policy, the director of the district media program seeks to create procedure specifications that provide appropriate quality controls and promote efficiency in purchasing. Bid policies permit rejection of any item bid that does not meet performance and service standards.

Items of equipment and production supplies, such as audiotape, videotape, film stock, and the like, can be purchased with a greater cost savings, in most instances, through a bid procedure. The procedure provides for acquisition of quality supplies and equipment by careful preparation of specifications that clearly define necessary electronic and mechanical requirements. Evaluations of equipment provided by the Educational Products Information Exchange Institute,[2] the *Library Technology Reports* of the American Library

1. Daniel Melcher, *Melcher on Acquisition* (Chicago: American Library Assn., 1971), p. 46.
2. *Educational Product Report* (Educational Products Information Exchange Institute, 463 West St., New York, NY 10014). 9 issues per yr., Oct.–June.

Association,[3] and other consumer testing programs should be considered in developing specifications. The bid procedure recognizes that cost savings are dependent not only upon initial price but also upon educational effectiveness, reliability, and ease of maintenance. Guarantees and the availability of warranty services are considered.

Production

Media production services provide for the preparation of materials not available from other sources and for the creation of materials by students or other users to enhance self-discovery and expression. Materials are produced in print, visual, auditory, and tactile formats for individual use, for presentations, and for small and large group activities. Uses of locally produced media range from a single application to incorporation of these materials into the district or school collection.

GUIDING PRINCIPLES

1. Local production of materials is performed at both district and individual school levels. The district production program both gives leadership to and complements production at the individual school level.
2. Production of materials not available from other sources is emphasized.
3. The production program supports the curriculum and applies knowledge of teaching/learning processes.
4. The goal of production is to match format to message.
5. The production program provides for the design and creation of materials by students and teachers, as well as by the media staff.
6. Policies for the production program recognize copyright laws and guard against their violation.
7. Production procedures insure that user requests are met promptly and efficiently.

3. *Library Technology Reports* (American Library Assn.). Bimonthly.

DISTRICT PRODUCTION PROGRAM

The district media program gives priority to producing materials not readily available from other sources or those which can be produced more economically or with greater adaptability. It extends the production capabilities (facilities, equipment, and staff competencies) available in most individual schools. Materials are designed and produced for teacher and student use, staff development activities, and public information purposes.

The scope and extent of district production is influenced by several factors: emphasis on production in individual schools, facilities and personnel at the district level, and the availability and use of specific production components, such as television and radio production or printing services, from sources outside the district.

Consideration is given to provision of the following types of district production services:

Graphics: graphics production staff prepares visuals for use in curriculum, staff development programs, presentations made by administrative and supervisory personnel, and public information programs.

Printing: production includes such materials as courses of study, resource units, catalogs of district media collections available to schools, and study guides accompanying locally produced television and radio programming, sound slide presentations, and other instructional materials.

Photography: still photography operations include photographing and developing black-and-white prints and photographing 2″ x 2″ slides. Motion picture photography includes production of Super 8mm films and 16mm films; alternatively, the district may contract for film production. District motion photography services extend the capabilities of individual schools and give support to student production of motion films.

Television and radio: the program provides or contracts with other agencies for the production of instructional television and radio programs and provides consultative and technical assistance to individual schools in television production activities. District services also provide for reception and videotape recording of educational telecasts needed for reuse in instruction, as permitted by copyright laws. Television programs recorded on video formats are made available for distribution in the schools by rebroadcast and/or by distribution of videotapes.

Audiotape production: the program produces audiotape recordings and copies audiotapes (in keeping with copyright regulations) by use of high-speed reel–to–reel and cassette tape duplicators.

Kits, models, and displays: production includes the designing of kits, models, learning activity packages, and displays tailored to local instructional needs. Commercial and locally produced materials can be combined in various formats.

District media program production services give emphasis to staff development programs, consultative help, and technical assistance in implementing school-based production programs. They provide leadership and guidance in media production activities by students and teachers, and, when beneficial, arrange for transportation of students to district media production centers offering capabilities not available in individual schools.

Channels of communication between district and school media staffs serve to identify quality productions developed by staff and/or students within one school which are of potential value to others. Provisions are made for sharing and/or duplicating such productions with due regard to the rights and privileges of individual authors or inventors.

SCHOOL PRODUCTION PROGRAM

The school media program is concerned with production by the media staff, teachers, aides, students, and even parents. It encourages the creation, adaption, and duplication of materials needed by teachers and students not readily or economically available elsewhere. The media staff provides and maintains convenient work areas, engages in production, and gives consultative and technical assistance to production projects.

Types of production are similar to many district production components but are typically less comprehensive in scope and less complex and sophisticated in technological capabilities. When practical, a production activity in a given format may be centered at an individual school for its own or for multischool use; for example, a large school may make extensive use of closed-circuit television programming or a vocational-technical high school may offer an advanced printing-trades curriculum. A school with a technician skillful in producing working models may offer to share these capabilities, while schools with learning programs that stress manual dexterities may offer a variety of production services, especially to elementary schools.

The school media program provides the following production capabilities, as a minimum:

> *Graphics*: the preparation of visuals, including dry mounting, laminating, and transparency production
> *Photography*: facilities and equipment for black-and-white photography, 2" x 2" color slides, and silent 8mm motion film photography
> *Television and radio*: the production of videotape recordings
> *Audiotape production*: the recording and duplicating of audiotapes.

Insofar as maturity levels permit, all facilities, equipment, supplies, and professional and technical assistance are available for student use. Student production occurs as a natural component of the educational experience and develops capabilities to translate elements of the environment into meaningful modes of communication. Creating materials in all formats sharpens the student's critical response to media, expands dialogue and the transmission of ideas, and fosters growth in precise and effective written and oral expression.

Budgeting for the school media program includes provisions for the equipment and supplies necessary for the production of materials. Listings of supplies required for production processes are not provided in this publication since the information is readily available in other sources. Enumeration of equipment requirements is limited to identification of basic types and levels of equipment for various processes.

Table 2 indicates school production capabilities. These are placed on a continuum that ranges from static forms through sound to motion which should be available to all users through the resources of the school media program, complemented as needed by resources available from the district media program.

Access and Delivery Systems

Access and delivery systems are the means by which students and teachers obtain materials, equipment, and other resources at the time of need or desire. Each system must have structure and definition, but creative organization and skill in making special adaptations are also basic to every operation. The best access and delivery systems require the least conscious conformity by the user.

GUIDING PRINCIPLES

1. Processing services provide efficient acquisition and organization of materials for accessibility to users.
2. Retrieval systems, e.g., cataloging, indexing, and remote access retrieval, facilitate use of all information in the school and district collections.
3. Access to information sources beyond the school and the district is provided by such means as cooperative arrangements with community agencies.
4. Principles of cost-effectiveness are used in determining the best level(s) and location(s)—classroom, school media center, district, or other—at which to provide media for various purposes.
5. Access to a variety of materials gives the user opportunity to grow in ability to make choices, compare ideas, and discover new interests.
6. The media program provides opportunities for the student to learn how to make self-directed searches for knowledge.

7. The test of any delivery system is how well it provides convenient, flexible, and speedy access to all media.

DISTRICT MEDIA PROGRAM

Decisions relative to access and delivery systems for the school district are the responsibility of the district media program director who also plans for suitable implementation. Heads of school media programs are oriented to and concerned with overall operations and contribute input to aid in evaluating their effectiveness.

Processing services include ordering, receiving, cataloging, physical processing, and distributing materials and equipment to the individual schools that selected them. Centralized accounting services are a desirable accompaniment. Processing services handle the acquisition and appropriate preparation of all types of formats—print, visual, auditory, and tactile—and accompanying equipment. The extent of processing varies with different formats; for example, processing services for periodicals and newspapers may be limited to acquisitions and accounting, textbooks receive simpler treatment than trade books, and equipment receives less physical processing than do materials.

Processing alternatives include provision of centralized processing at the district level; contracting for processing services that are available from a multidistrict, regional, or state center; use of commercial processing; and combinations of these approaches. Handling of processing at the individual school level is rarely advisable in terms of economy and efficiency. In determining the system or combination of systems that best meet the district's need, consideration is given to size of the operation, number and proportions of different formats to be processed, number of duplicate items, available personnel, available space, existing studies comparing costs of commercial services with typical district-operated services, available funds, and any constraints upon uses of these funds.

Districts which decide to use commercial processing services need to supplement these services by providing centralized acquisitions and receipt, cataloging and processing for materials and equipment now not available from commercial services, and cataloging and processing for locally produced materials.

TABLE 2.   SCHOOL PRODUCTION CAPABILITIES

| FORMAT | BASIC COMPONENTS | | ADVANCED COMPONENTS | | DISPLAY TECHNOLOGY |
	PROCESS	EQUIPMENT	PROCESS	EQUIPMENT	
Puppet Productions 3-Dimensional Construction	Commercial Hand-sewing Construction	Tools & art materials			Puppet theater Record player Tape recorder
Printing	Hand-lettering Copying Illustrating	Typewriter Spirit duplicator Mimeograph	Preparation of masters Typesetting Layout	Press(es) 8" x 10" copy camera Equipped darkroom	
Overhead Transparencies	Direct: Write-on Painted Hand-embellished Thermal Color lift	Thermal copier Laminator	Diazo Photographic	Diazo printer & developer 8" x 10" copy camera Equipped darkroom	Overhead projector
Flat Pictures and Posters	Hand-drawing Dry mounting	Dry mount press & tacking iron	Photographic	Cameras Equipped darkroom	Opaque projector Display areas
Slides and Filmstrips	Direct: Write-on Painted Slides Photographic	Simple slide-format camera w/copy stand	Filmstrips, photographic Slides, photographic Sound slides & filmstrips	35mm half-frame camera w/appropriate accessories 35mm single-reflex camera Recorder w/synchronizer	Slide projector Slide viewer Filmstrip projector Filmstrip viewer Tape recorder w/synchronizer

TABLE 2 (*continued*).

| FORMAT | BASIC COMPONENTS | | ADVANCED COMPONENTS | | DISPLAY TECHNOLOGY |
	PROCESS	EQUIPMENT	PROCESS	EQUIPMENT	
Audiotape Recordings	Reel-to-reel Cassette	Reel-to-reel tape recorder Cassette tape recorder		Soundproof room Audiomixer with monaural & stereo capability	Reel-to-reel tape recorder Cassette tape recorder
Motion Picture Production	Direct: painted Photographic: silent	Super 8mm camera	Photographic, sound	Camera w/sound capability (may use recorder) 16mm camera Film editor	Super 8mm projector 16mm projector Tape recorder
Multi-image Presentations	(May combine any or all of the above processes & equipment)		(May combine any or all of the above processes & equipment)		Projection equipment Programmer Dissolve unit
Television Productions	Videotape recording Off-the-air One or two camera operation	Videotape recorder ½″ or ¾″ 1–2 video cameras Switcher, video & audio	Studio productions	Equipped studio Appropriate VTR Film chain Switcher, video & audio	Videotape recorder Monitor
Computer Programming			Audio Printed Visual Any combination of above	Keyboard & appropriate computer programming equipment	Computer terminal Display system

Processing organizes materials and equipment to make them more accessible to the user. Uniform, high quality cataloging that is curriculum- and user-oriented is the objective, with operations performed in order to extend the time available for school media specialists to work with users and to minimize the cost and time requirements for processing services. The district's provisions for processing services insure that initial collections are ready for use in new schools when they open, that collections are processed for both individual school and district level collections, and that data are collected for related purposes such as compiling special bibliographies.

Other district media program functions that promote access to information sources include coordinating development of community resource files, developing policies that facilitate school use of community resources, coordinating telecommunications activities within the district, and investigating and arranging for districtwide participation in larger-area (multidistrict, regional, state) media programs that afford extended access to broader media resources. Provisions for access to resources beyond those of the school and the district require clearly defined policies and procedures.

District media program operations, such as processing services, equipment services, film and videotape collections, and the like, are supported by convenient delivery systems for frequent pickup and delivery of materials and equipment among schools and the district center.

SCHOOL MEDIA PROGRAM

The school media program seeks to provide prompt and efficient access to the resources of the school media program—program, staff, facilities, and collections—for teachers and students. One of the best means for achieving this goal is flexible scheduling, rather than scheduling that preempts facilities and staff for fixed periods of time assigned over a semester or year. Open scheduling permits access by individuals and small groups at the time of need or interest and provides opportunities for teachers to schedule groups of students to the media center for specific purposes. Use of the media center as an assigned study hall is educationally indefensible. The media center is available before, throughout, and after regular school hours, with consideration given to extended hours of operation, as warranted by the needs of teachers and learners.

Schools develop delivery systems that make media more easily obtainable. With dial access the computer enables users to have immediate access to print, aural, and visual materials through the facilities of their carrels. Remote access systems perform in less sophisticated but effective ways. A central area responds to user requests made usually by telephone or an intercom system, and the tape, film, or filmstrip operated in the central area is heard or seen in the carrel.

The total concept of access extends beyond dissemination of the school collection and includes interinstitutional loans and cooperation with other information sources such as the public library, academic libraries, museums, and art galleries. Further, it draws upon the agencies and services of the community, setting up interviews, arranging visits to businesses and industries, and providing systems of idea exchange with students of other schools. Such activities are all part of the access and delivery operations of the media program.

Materials and portable equipment are circulated from the media center for use throughout the school and in the home. It offers a variety of alternatives in media formats and activities, encouraging free exploration of available resources. The tendency to isolate from general use materials and equipment in classroom storage should be avoided. When both teachers and students draw upon the media center for items such as puzzles, kits, and other types of learning resources, the overall use of these materials substantially increases. Borrowing may be in the form of long-term loans for classroom use.

The head of the school media program works with the administration and the teachers in defining policies for student use of the media center, emphasizing student analysis, comparison, and the critical evaluation of sources. Guidance in self-directed search for information is provided to aid in expanded and more effective uses of information sources. The media staff draws upon the expertise provided by their training and experience to enable learners to acquire research skills and reading, viewing, and listening techniques that enhance their ability to select and use media. This is a special and unique contribution that media professionals make to students at every maturity level.

53

Maintenance

Maintenance calls for diverse operations. It extends from cords of projectors and spines of books to nonfunctioning projectors and tape recorders. Its purposes are dual—good maintenance contributes largely to the comfort and efficiency of learners, teachers, and staff; it also plays an important part in economical and efficient management.

GUIDING PRINCIPLES

1. Preventive maintenance insures longer life of materials and equipment.
2. All types of materials and equipment are inspected periodically to prevent, detect, and repair damage.
3. Budget provisions are made for replacement of worn materials unsuitable for repair and of items of equipment for which maintenance costs exceed replacement costs.

The appearance of district media program areas and school media centers at all times reflects good long-range maintenance and day-by-day care. Provision for adequate maintenance and upkeep does not require the services of media professionals.

The collection of materials and equipment is always in good condition; items within it are competently maintained, inviting to use, and immediately ready.

Media staff perform preventive maintenance by such tasks as reinforcing and repairing materials, changing lamps and fuses, and regularly inspecting and cleaning equipment. Users are encouraged to report any damages or malfunctions they observe. To avoid both the necessity for repairs and the possibility of user frustrations, items requiring special precautions are identified by such labels as *Do Not Bend, Do Not Move Projector While Lamp Is On,* and the like. Instruction in use of materials and equipment emphasizes proper handling and care of collections.

Continuous checking of the condition of materials and equipment within the collection is an established part of the circulation system. In addition, systematic inspection is scheduled at regular intervals.

Records of equipment usage and maintenance provide data for analyzing the cost-effectiveness of given items, and the district media director creates such forms or directs the heads of school media programs in setting up record-keeping systems. These records are used as a basis for making decisions to replace items of equipment for which repair costs become excessive.

The head of the school media program plans maintenance procedures according to the policies of the district media program and the services it provides for major repairing and reconditioning of equipment. The school administration is knowledgeable of these procedures.

The media program budget provides funds approximating 3 percent of the total inventory value (replacement cost) of equipment for use in purchasing replacement parts. It is recommended that the district media program assume the costs of providing replacement lamps, fuses, and similar items for individual schools.

Public Information

Public information is the communications process by which the media staff provides and transmits information about media program objectives and functions to develop public awareness and support.

GUIDING PRINCIPLES

1. Goals for the public information program are established through the planning process and reflect understanding of the various audiences to be reached.
2. Satisfaction of user needs is the most essential component of effective public relations.
3. Public information and public relations are considered in all areas of media program operations and are provided on a continuing basis.
4. The public information program provides for coordinated exchange of information with other agencies at district, regional, state, and national levels.
5. Provisions for collection and analysis of data on the media program are based on the utility of the data

for program evaluation and public information purposes.
6. Public information is recognized as an effective tool
in assuring intellectual freedom for users.

The program of public information is a major means of achieving
the objectives of the media program, and its goals are developed
through the planning process. Audiences reached by this program
include student and teacher users, administrators at the school and
district levels, parents, the board of education, and the general public including audiences beyond the local community. It provides
appropriate information for each audience group, geared to its needs
and conveyed in the most effective manner.

Teachers and students should know the ways in which the media
program can help them achieve learning objectives. Administrators
need to know how the media program functions in relation to other
components of the educational system, and they require supporting
data for budget and planning purposes. Parents should understand
the relationships among media, instructional design, and the curriculum. The board of education reflects and influences community attitudes through its priorities, explanations, and budgets. The general
public is concerned with both the effectiveness and the efficiency of
the educational program.

A well-planned program of public relations interprets the role of
the media program and extends public expectations. Satisfied users
of a media program are a crucial link in the public information system. Staff development programs offer significant opportunities to
extend teachers' knowledge of and competence in using media.
Consultative work with administrators and consultants in using media for public information purposes, plus production of materials for
such presentations, promotes broader recognition of the role of
media in the total educational program.

Public information programs have a responsibility for protecting
intellectual freedom in the media program. Sharing goals and objectives with the community and soliciting input in return provide a
rational basis for decision-making and reasonable interchange in
times of philosophic disagreement.

The director of the district media program has general responsibility for planning the public information program, working with

TABLE 3. RECOMMENDATIONS FOR AN EFFECTIVE PUBLIC INFORMATION PROGRAM

AUDIENCE	TYPES OF INFORMATION NEEDED	MEANS FOR PROVIDING INFORMATION
Students	Media center resources and program functions Ways of using media in reaching educational objectives Contributions of media to personal interests and goals	Displays, posters, news releases Media production Media presentations Personal contact Classroom visits Indirect contact through teachers Bibliographies Media packages
School Staff (faculty and administrators)	Media program goals and functions Ways of using media to achieve educational objectives Role of media in the total educational program Use of media to reach personal and professional goals	Memoranda, handbooks, information sheets Personal contacts and conferences Staff meetings Staff development programs on media utilization News releases Media production Media presentations Bibliographies Annual reports
Parents, Citizens, Board of Education, Other Public Officials	Media program goals and functions and their role in the achievement of overall educational goals Media program operations in relationship to the total educational program	News releases, radio and television coverage Media presentations Personal contacts Open house programs, public exhibits Budget justifications Annual reports
Media and Education Agencies and Associations	Media program goals and functions Program plans and activities as they relate to other agencies	News releases Annual reports Information sheets and handbooks Personal contact Participation in association activities Contribution to professional publications

district and school media staff members and with the school district public information officer. A process for the exchange of views and ideas insures continuous participation by individual schools.

The head of the school media program develops and coordinates public information activities at the individual school level. Information for students depends on their maturity level, but unless they are kept informed they do not develop proprietary interests in the media program. Information to teachers helps to establish the professional rapport necessary for effective instructional design. Public information to parents eases and improves the use of media out of school.

Data collection by the district media program and individual school programs is closely related to public information needs. The district media program director determines the types of information needed in terms of potential use and sets forth the means to be used in collecting, storing, and analyzing data. The heads of school media programs are oriented in and given the means to fulfill their part of the program. State and national guidelines are followed in collecting and reporting statistical information.

Audiences to be reached, types of information to be provided, and means for providing that information are outlined in table 3.

Program Evaluation

The purpose of evaluation is to assess the degree to which goals and objectives have been met and to determine the effectiveness of program elements in relation to their achievement. Such evaluation results in the continuation of a program element or its modification or discontinuance. Evaluation is the only professional basis for such decisions.

GUIDING PRINCIPLES

1. Effective planning for media program rests upon adequate evaluation of program elements and it yields information for program planning and improvement.
2. Evaluation is a continuous process, conducted at all levels (district and school), involving both staff and users of the media program.

3. The director of the district media program plans and coordinates internal evaluation of the media program at district and school levels and works with other district personnel in the planning for evaluation of the media program within the context of the total educational program.
4. In addition to continuing evaluation, in-depth evaluations of media program elements are made at periodic intervals.
5. Evaluations conducted by persons or groups outside the school district contribute additional information and insights for program improvement.

The media staff uses evaluation as an ongoing process by which to determine the effectiveness of the program in achieving stated objectives. The findings of evaluation are applied in planning for program modification, budgeting, staff deployment, collections development, and public information.

EVALUATION AT THE DISTRICT LEVEL

Primary responsibility for designing and implementing the evaluation plan rests at the district level. The director of the district media program coordinates planning for evaluation of the media program, and in doing so works with other media staff, district personnel who represent administration, curriculum, planning, research, and evaluation, and the heads of school media programs. The evaluation process also seeks input from users concerned with the program or program element being evaluated.

A comprehensive plan provides for:

Evaluation of the media program in the context of the total educational program—incorporated in evaluation of the total educational program of the district or of a specific program area

Ongoing evaluation of district media program components and individual school media programs by media staff and users

Periodic evaluation, in depth, of the total media program or specific components

Special evaluation projects conducted by outside evaluators, offering a more objective view of the program and expert advice from recognized outside consultants

Combined internal/external evaluation, which characterizes programs for school accreditation.

EVALUATION AT THE SCHOOL LEVEL

Within the school media center program, the head of the school media program institutes the same types of evaluation with the same purposes as the director of the district media program. The heads of school media programs are in constant contact with the director of the district program and their school administrators in seeking to perfect evaluation instruments, to interpret them properly, and to apply their findings to program modifications.

The school media program seeks information consonant to its role within the school. It evaluates such concerns as:

Extent of the school population it reaches

Level of participation by teachers and learners

Effectiveness of its leadership and its cooperative efforts in instructional design and its implementation

Ability to establish priorities with the school administration that result in sufficient budget for materials and equipment, and the way that these funds are allocated

Extent of cooperation with other media programs and community agencies

Satisfactions, rewards, and growth of the school media staff

Role of the school media program in total community efforts for children and youth.

Application of findings obtained through evaluation result in improved instructional design. These findings identify the means for improving learning environments that permit learners to work independently and in teams on tasks they help to design, for which they search out essential resources and which they assess for effectiveness.

Within the framework of curriculum objectives, good evaluation increasingly enables students to exercise control over what they are to learn and to assume responsibility for deciding how they will achieve their goals.

Improved educational opportunities occur when learners are expected to assess how effectively they are using resources: people and organizations; content in print, visual, tactile, and auditory formats; self-instructional materials; and raw materials and equipment useful for translating ideas into meaningful communication. Such objectivity extends user satisfaction and builds a sense of personal significance in the learning process. The student grows in abilities to set goals and to revise them as progress occurs; to recognize, use, and improve various learning modes; and to work with numerous and diverse information sources.

Evaluations of experiences and assessments of materials and processes by students and teachers are integral parts of the school media program. They are sought by the media staff and they contribute to the ongoing cycle of development and renewal, providing needed assurances for the media professionals who strive to achieve program goals and objectives.

6 Collections

Strong media collections provide the primary means for teaching, learning, and interest fulfillment. A school's media collection represents the essential informational base of the instructional program. Media professionals contribute expertise in evaluating and selecting materials and equipment to the process of building and maintaining adequate collections.

GUIDING PRINCIPLES

1. Every school, regardless of size, has its own collection of materials and equipment. This collection, which is organized and ready for use when the school opens, is developed and expanded on a planned basis.
2. The district provides collections of materials and equipment, such as 16mm films, professional materials, and examination collections of new materials, to supplement collections in the individual schools.
3. Selection of collections is guided by a selection policy formulated by media staff, administrators, consultants, teachers, students, and representative citizens, and adopted by the board of education. The district policy is supplemented by selection and acquisitions guidelines formulated by individual schools within the district.
4. Selection of materials is a cooperative process involving the media staff, curriculum consultants, teachers, students, and community representatives and is coordinated by the director of the district media program and the head of the school media program respectively.

5. Materials and equipment are evaluated prior to purchase by use of reliable evaluative selection tools
and by firsthand examination, wherever possible.
6. Collections are reevaluated continuously to insure
that they remain current and responsive to user
needs.
7. Organization and arrangement make the collection
easily accessible to users.
8. Materials in print, visual, auditory, and tactile formats, with associated equipment, constitute the collection.
9. Collections include textbooks and related instructional materials and systems.
10. Current professional materials for faculty and staff
use are a part of the collection.

School media personnel assume responsibility for insuring that
users have ready access to the materials and equipment they need
or want. Ready and convenient access is the essence of media program development, matching interests or desires with one or more
of a broad range of media, with confidence in the power generated
by the union of user and material. The special training and skills of
media personnel provide leadership in building a relevant, diverse
collection, in making it accessible, and in supplying services that
enhance the quality of participants' experiences as they relate their
involvement in media to their own fulfillment.

The user's first point of convenient access to materials is the
media center in his own school. No substitute can replace the individual school collection in guaranteeing a high degree of user satisfaction, but it is unrealistic to claim that any school can provide
within its own walls all of the materials and equipment that users
need. The media staff takes the initiative in obtaining needed information and material from other sources, using interlibrary loans
from other schools, school district media collections, local public
libraries, college and university libraries, and regional, state, and
national networks.

Sharing of materials between schools is a cooperative venture.
Leadership emanates from the district media program, but cooperative approaches in collections development rest upon joint planning

in which each participating school assumes responsibility for building strong collections in specific subject areas and/or for developing specified holdings of periodicals and pamphlets in microform editions, with accompanying provisions for sharing these materials with other schools.

Identification and organization of information on available community resources, both human and material, is another approach by which users' needs are satisfied.

Selection Policies and Procedures

Formulation of a district media selection policy which guides the selection of materials and equipment is coordinated by the director of the district media program. This policy, developed cooperatively with representation of media staff, administrators, consultants, teachers, students, and other community members, is adopted by the board of education as official district policy.

The media selection policy reflects basic factors influencing the nature and scope of collections, such as curriculum trends, innovations in instruction, research in learning, availability of materials and equipment, the increased sophistication of youth, and the rising expectations of teachers and students. It establishes the objectives of media selection; identifies personnel participating in selection and their roles; enumerates types of materials and equipment to be considered with criteria for their evaluation, as well as criteria for evaluating materials in specific subject areas; and defines procedures followed in selecting materials, including initial selection, reexamination of titles in existing collections, and handling challenged titles.

The selection policy reflects and supports principles of intellectual freedom described in the *Library Bill of Rights*,[1] the *School Library Bill of Rights for School Library Media Center Programs*,[2] *The Students' Right to Read*,[3] and other professional statements on in-

1. The *Library Bill of Rights* was adopted by the Council of the American Library Association in 1948 and amended in 1961 and 1967.

2. The *School Library Bill of Rights for School Library Media Center Programs* was approved by the American Association of School Librarians in 1969.

3. National Council of Teachers of English, *The Students' Right to Read* (Urbana, Ill.: National Council of Teachers of English, 1972).

tellectual freedom. Procedures for handling questioned materials follow established guidelines and are clearly defined.[4]

The district selection policy is supplemented by selection and acquisitions guidelines formulated by each school which provide more detailed and specific guidance for building and maintaining the school's collections.

Basic to effective selection is the establishment of cooperatively developed priorities that consider the existing collection and identify its strengths, gaps, and pertinency. Selection of materials involves the media staff, administrators, curriculum consultants, teachers, and students, with the process coordinated by the head of the school media program.

Building a collection calls for careful planning; understanding of the school program and the interests, abilities, and problems of the population; broad current knowledge of materials available and the related equipment; and an understanding of the district selection policy and budgeting procedures. It also requires objective judgments, discriminating taste, and a sensitivity to the needs and concerns of learners and teachers. Continuous reassessment, both of the program priorities and the appropriateness of the collection, insures an adequate response to changing programs, populations, and opportunities.

Examination and Evaluation of Media

The process of examining and evaluating materials and equipment being considered for purchase is continuous and systematic. The district media program supports the selection process by providing examination collections of materials and equipment, arranging for released time for preview and examination of materials, and conducting an active evaluation program involving media personnel, teachers, other staff, and students. Published evaluations, including those in reviews, recommended lists, and standard bibliographic tools are used in selection. Materials and equipment within existing collections are monitored and examined continuously in order to replace worn items and to withdraw out-of-date and inappropriate items.

4. "Intellectual Freedom and School Libraries; An In-Depth Case Study," *School Media Quarterly*, 1:111–35 (Winter 1973).

DISTRICT COLLECTIONS

The school district through the district media program provides for individual schools additional materials or equipment which meet one or more of the following criteria:

Too expensive for each school to afford in sufficient quantity, i.e., 16mm films

Infrequently used

Rare, e.g., certain specimens and museum objects not available in duplicate

Needed on a temporary basis, e.g., equipment to replace school-owned equipment being repaired

Provided for examination and consideration for purchase, e.g., new materials and equipment included in a district educational media selection center.

FILMS, VIDEOTAPES, AND RELATED COLLECTIONS. Through its own collection or through participation in a multidistrict film library program, the district media program provides access for individual schools to at least 3,000 titles, with sufficient duplicate prints to satisfy 90 percent of all requests. This is a minimal figure and access to additional titles up to a total of 5,000 titles may be needed. In addition, sufficient funds are provided for purchase and/or rental of new and specialized titles as needed throughout the year. Selection of materials in 16mm or video format is based on quality of image, utilization mode, size of intended viewing audience, availability of materials and equipment, and cost of changeover from one format to the other.

PROFESSIONAL MATERIALS. The district professional library gives administrators, curriculum consultants, teachers, media professionals, and other district and school staff convenient access to professional materials by which to keep informed of trends, developments, techniques, research, and experimentation in general and specialized areas of education. It includes works in such related subjects as communications, sociology, anthropology, behavioral psychology, the humanities, linguistics, and philosophy. Information sources may include books and pamphlets, government documents, journals, films, filmstrips, videotapes, and audiotapes. The collection of professional materials provided at the district level is complemented by smaller, working collections in individual schools.

The professional library also includes the following types of resources:

Curriculum materials, including courses of study, curriculum guides, resource units, and teacher's manuals

Selection tools that index, evaluate, and review instructional materials

Television and radio program guides and manuals

Indexes of community resources including catalogs and brochures of sites of educational value and field trip evaluations

Information on teachers' organizations and associations, forthcoming meetings, and programs for continuing education.

MEDIA SELECTION AND EVALUATION CENTER. The district media program supports the selection of materials and equipment by individual school media programs by providing examination collections of materials and equipment, arranging for released time for school personnel to preview and examine materials, and conducting an active evaluation program that involves media personnel, teachers, curriculum consultants, and other users.

The media selection center staff facilitates the evaluation process through these activities:

Collection and organization of materials for examination

Capture and dissemination of published evaluations of media

Development and provision of improved criteria and data forms to gather responses from users

Arranging for user evaluations (assignment of persons and media, assistance and guidance)

Collecting and organizing the resulting data and dissemination of the findings on a timely basis.[5]

5. Cora Paul Bomar, M. Ann Heidbreder, and Carol A. Nemeyer, *Guide to the Development of Educational Media Selection Centers* (ALA Studies in Librarianship, no. 4 [Chicago: American Library Assn., 1973]), p. 30.

SCHOOL COLLECTIONS

The collection in each school is rich in breadth and depth of content and represents varied types of materials, points of view, and forms of expression. It provides a broad range of media formats and meets the requirements of all curriculum areas, accommodating diverse learning skills and styles of users at varying maturity and ability levels.

Funds provided for media center collections are sufficient to enable the school media program to meet accepted standards for the collection, secure additional materials and equipment needed for changing curricula and student populations, and maintain the collection in satisfactory condition.

Capital outlay funds provided for new schools establish initial collections ready for use when the school opens. Allocations in addition to the usual operating funds are essential to expand collections in new and reorganized schools. Higher than average per pupil allocations are required for schools with small enrollments, changing needs, or special programs that require extensive materials and resources.

The primary factors in building a school media collection are the requirements of the instructional program and the needs and interests of users. Budgeting practices provide for flexibility in the choice of media formats, with proper relationships between collections, staff requirements, and physical facilities, particularly space required for the use and storage of materials and equipment, rationally derived. Other considerations include the packaging or repackaging of items to increase durability, the assembling of kits of materials that complement or enhance each other, and the transferring of content from one format to another.

A single model for the collection of materials and equipment is not presented here, since decisions concerning amounts of materials, their formats, and quantities of supporting equipment are made on the basis of program and user needs. However, these guidelines do identify base quantities of materials and associated equipment needed to insure adequate provisions for content coverage, range in levels, and choice of media formats, responding to general information needs and personal interests and preferences.

It is recommended that a school with 500 or fewer students have a minimum collection of 20,000 items or 40 per student. An item is defined as a book (casebound or paperback), film, videotape, filmstrip, transparency, slide, periodical subscription, kit, any other form of material, or associated equipment. It is possible that the collection in larger schools may provide the needed range in content, levels, forms of expression, and formats at a ratio of less than 40 items per student.

Recommendations recognize the need to obtain materials and equipment that supplement items provided within the individual school. Access to additional collections is recommended and can be achieved only through arrangements designed to guarantee availability of a broader choice of media, as, for example, planning for the school population to use a public library which offers breadth and depth in collections. Cooperative relationships that prescribe both the means by which to implement interlibrary loans and the measure of the adequacy of such provisions are essential. Similarly, planning for the use of any community, school district, or multi-district resource should include adequate guarantees for a high degree of satisfaction of users' needs.

The recommended base collection for the media program in the individual school, with accompanying suggestions for achieving excellence in meeting user needs, follows. The total number of items in the lower range is less than the recommended minimum of 20,000 items, while the total number in the higher range is greater. Final decisions about the mix of materials, including actual quantities in each category, are made in the individual school. The development of the media collection is based on program goals and characteristics of the school and reflects needs, prior action, and resources. The recommendations which follow provide a continuum leading to excellence in meeting student needs.

Collections: Recommendations for Meeting
User Needs

BASE COLLECTION IN THE SCHOOL	EXTENDED PROVISIONS

Note: Base recommendations are presented for a school with 500 or fewer users, and represent items located within the school.

Note: Recommendations for access to collections beyond the school call for planned arrangements that guarantee a high degree of user satisfaction.

TOTAL COLLECTION
At least 20,000 items located in the school
or
40 items per user

There is no limit to potential user need and therefore no justifiable quantitative limit to the size of a collection. Beyond the recommended base, the budget permits expansion of the collection when needs arise.

The media staff obtains for users additional items available from local, regional, state, and federal agencies.

PRINT MATERIALS: Books, Periodicals and Newspapers, Pamphlets, Microforms

BOOKS

8,000 to 12,000 volumes
or
16 to 24 per user

Access to 60,000 titles to insure satisfaction of 90 percent of initial requests

Considerations in making choices:

1. The collection provides for subject, interest, and reference coverage, multiple reading and maturity levels in each subject area, and representation of varying points of view.
2. Titles are selected on the basis of such established elements of evaluation as appeal and value for users, accuracy, currency, style, and quality of format.
3. Sufficient duplication of titles is provided to satisfy user demands.
4. Paperback books are purchased to satisfy heavy demands for particular titles, to provide less-used titles in an inexpensive format, and to respond to user preferences.

BASE COLLECTION IN THE SCHOOL	EXTENDED PROVISIONS

PERIODICALS AND NEWSPAPERS

50 to 175 titles	Access to research capability in periodical/newspaper literature, by purchasing microform collections, by photocopying, and/or interlibrary loan

Considerations in making choices:

1. The collection supports the curriculum, caters to the interests of users, represents different points of view, provides intellectual and aesthetic stimulation, and responds to the professional needs of teachers.
2. Appropriate indexes are provided for magazine and newspaper holdings.
3. Magazines and newspapers that contribute to satisfaction of user needs are considered for acquisition although they may not be indexed.
4. Back issues of selected periodicals are readily available in the media center. Holdings that extend back more than five years are retained, discarded, or replaced by microform editions, according to needs.
5. Local, state, national, and international newspapers are represented in the collection.
6. Duplicate titles are provided for periodicals in heavy demand.

PAMPHLETS

The type and quantity vary according to program needs	Use of depository libraries provides access to extensive holdings of government documents

Considerations in making choices:

1. The collection includes state, national, and international government documents, which represent important sources of information.
2. Items in the collection are useful, current, and varied in points of view.
3. Persons or organizations responsible for the publication are clearly identified on items included in the collection.

71

BASE COLLECTION IN THE SCHOOL	EXTENDED PROVISIONS

4. Free and inexpensive materials, selected with care, are included as appropriate. Simplified order procedures permit rapid acquisition of free and inexpensive materials.
5. Much time and effort are required to maintain and index a clipping file; preferred alternatives include increasing periodical subscriptions and/or indexes and use of commercial clipping services, if needed.

MICROFORMS: MICROFILM, MICROCARD, AND MICROFICHE

Types and quantity vary with program needs.	User access to extensive microform data bases, e.g., Educational Resources Information Center (ERIC), Human Relations Area Files (HRAF), etc.
	Cooperative approaches among schools in collection-building, with accompanying arrangements for interlibrary loans and/or photocopying

MICROFORM EQUIPMENT: READERS AND PRINTERS

2 readers, 1 of which is portable, plus 1 reader-printer	Sufficient number of readers (portable and stationary) and reader-printers to satisfy user needs

Considerations in making choices:

1. Microforms are important sources for primary source materials, back issues of periodicals, and government documents.
2. Factors of use, need for subject matter, technical quality, and availability of equipment are considered in purchasing microforms.
3. Provisions for appropriate indexing, storage, and equipment are made to insure easy and dependable retrieval of items in microform formats.
4. Equipment selection is based on quality of image reproduction, ease of operation, and durability.
5. Both portable and stationary equipment is provided.

BASE COLLECTION IN THE SCHOOL	EXTENDED PROVISIONS

VISUAL MATERIALS: Still Images

FILMSTRIPS: SOUND AND SILENT

500 to 2,000 items or 1 to 4 items per user	Access to sufficient items to insure satisfaction of 90 percent of initial requests In individualized programs in which students work with this format, a collection of 5,000 items is recommended.

FILMSTRIP EQUIPMENT: SILENT AND SOUND PROJECTORS AND VIEWERS

10 projectors and 30 viewers	One projector per teacher and One viewer per three users

Considerations in making choices:

1. Filmstrips meet accepted criteria for accuracy and scope of content, organization, and technical qualities. In addition they have user appeal and are appropriate in treatment for the intended use, i.e., self-directed use or teacher presentation.
2. Sound filmstrips selected for the collection have appropriate relationships between visual and auditory content.
3. Packaging of the filmstrip(s) and related materials is convenient for effective use and storage. Choices between alternative formats for audio reproduction are based on the same considerations.
4. The relative emphasis given to sound versus silent projectors and viewers is based on the nature of the collection and predominant patterns of use.
5. Remote control attachments are provided to promote effective use and interaction in group settings.

SLIDES AND TRANSPARENCIES

2,000 to 6,000 items or 4 to 12 items per user	Access to 15,000 items, including specialized subject collections, as needed in relation to instructional and user interests

BASE COLLECTION IN THE SCHOOL	EXTENDED PROVISIONS

SLIDE AND TRANSPARENCY EQUIPMENT

Slide projectors: 6, or
1 for every 100 users
Slide viewers: 10, or
1 for every 50 users
Overhead projectors: 10,* or
1 for every 50 users

*Varies with type of instructional program (see no. 6 in the following list of considerations).

Sufficient slide projectors to satisfy user demands plus additional dissolve units and synchronizers for displays

Additional overhead projectors available on demand from the district media program

Considerations in making choices:

1. Slides and transparencies are evaluated carefully for accuracy and technical qualities, including color, mounting, and (in the case of art slides) fidelity to the original. Legibility for the viewer is essential.
2. High selectivity is exercised in the purchase of sets of transparency masters.
3. Locally produced slides and transparencies are added to the collection when they meet criteria for quality and need.
4. Appropriate storage for single slides and sets of slides is provided.
5. Overhead projectors selected for the collection provide a standard 10″ x 10″ aperture and provide a sharp and clearly focused projected image appropriate in size for the intended use.
6. The proportion of overhead projectors needed is higher in schools with instructional patterns that emphasize teacher lecture and lower in schools that emphasize individualized and independent study approaches.
7. In the selection of slide projection equipment, care is taken to choose appropriate automatic slide projectors together with the most compatible and standardized dissolve units, synchronizers, and programming units. Choices made insure both design capability to do the job needed and ease in accomplishing it.
8. Remote control devices, as well as lenses of appropriate focal length, are acquired for slide projectors.
9. Selected slide viewers use slide trays compatible with those used with slide projectors.

GRAPHICS: POSTERS, ART AND STUDY PRINTS, MAPS AND GLOBES

800 to 1,200 items   Additional items to respond to program needs, with provision for original art, children's art, and loans of circulating collections from museums

Considerations in making choices:

1. Fidelity of reproduction to original artwork, including sharp focus and accurate color, is essential in collections of posters and art prints.
2. The collection includes examples of varied reproduction processes.
3. Items within a set of posters or prints are evaluated individually in order to determine the contribution and impact of the set as a whole.
4. Selection of maps and globes takes into account such factors as the following:

   True sizes and relationships of hemispheres are represented only through globes

   The larger the globe size, the greater the detail that can be shown

   Illumination of globes is minimally preferable

   Topographic and road maps of local areas are included in the collection

   Some maps may be provided in alternative formats, e.g., transparencies and microforms.

5. Criteria applied in evaluation of maps and globes include currency of features; appropriateness of scale; quality of drafting, engraving, and printing; clearly executed design that avoids confused appearance; clear typefaces.
6. Consideration is given to appropriate processing and storage of materials in fragile formats by such means as laminating, mounting, or framing items.

| BASE COLLECTION IN THE SCHOOL | EXTENDED PROVISIONS |

VISUAL MATERIALS: Moving Images

16MM AND SUPER 8MM SOUND FILMS, VIDEOTAPES, AND TELEVISION RECEPTION

Access to a minimum of 3,000 titles, with sufficient duplicate prints to satisfy 90 percent of all requests

In addition, sufficient funds for rental of specialized films, including feature-length films, when needed

Availability of sufficient funds throughout the year to provide for purchase and/or rental of new and specialized titles, on demand

Access to additional titles up to a total of 5,000 titles, from district film library, may be desirable

16MM AND SUPER 8MM SOUND PROJECTION AND VIDEO PLAYBACK AND RECEPTION EQUIPMENT

6 units, with 2 assigned to the media center
   plus
1 additional unit for each 100 users

The mix of 16mm and Super 8mm sound projectors and video playback and reception units depends upon the availability of materials in each format

Additional units to satisfy use by students, individually and in small groups, and for home use

Ratio of 1 unit per 50 users

Considerations in making choices:

1. Selection of 16mm or Super 8mm sound film or video (open-reel, cassette, and cartridge) format is based on consideration of quality of image, utilization mode, size of viewing audience, availability of materials and equipment, and cost of changeover from one format to the other.
2. Centralized collections of materials provided at the district (or multidistrict) level supply materials in sufficient depth to satisfy 90 percent of users' requests.
3. To serve the needs of film study programs, collections include frequently used feature films acquired on a long-term loan or purchase basis and/or make provisions for obtaining such films through a cooperative rental program.
4. 16mm film prints used six or more times a year in an individual school merit consideration for purchase.

5. Collections include materials produced by students and staff that meet criteria for quality and need.
6. Acquisition of Super 8mm sound films and projectors is based on careful evaluation of capability to reproduce sound and availability of appropriate materials and equipment.
7. Satisfactory condition of materials is assured by a maintenance and distribution system that checks, rewinds, cleans, and repairs each item after use.
8. Collections are evaluated continuously to identify materials requiring replacement and to withdraw obsolete items.
9. Equipment selection emphasizes adequacy and reliability of equipment and availability of servicing and repair, as well as availability of spare parts.
10. Selection of video playback and reception equipment provides for standardization of formats, to facilitate development of collections of video materials.
11. Video playback equipment is selected to provide for maximum simplicity and error-free operation with a minimum of controls.
12. Selection of 16mm projectors is based on specific criteria related to the intended use of the equipment. Choice between self-threading and manual-threading projectors takes into account convenience of use and ease of operation.
13. Each school acquires at least one 16mm projector with stop-motion (still frame) mechanism.
14. It is desirable, especially for the use of feature films, to provide for location of the projector's speaker close to the projection screen. Such provision can be made by use of an extension speaker or by installation of specialized wiring systems for remote sound.
15. For auditorium projection, a projector with a high intensity light source is desirable.

SUPER 8MM FILMS, SILENT

500 to 1,000 items
or
1 to 2 per user

Access to 4,000 titles from the individual school's collection, other schools, and a supplementary collection at the district level

BASE COLLECTION IN THE SCHOOL	EXTENDED PROVISIONS
	Development of specialized subject collections to be shared by individual schools is recommended

Super 8mm equipment

20 cartridge-loaded projectors and sufficient open-reel projectors to accommodate use of available films plus 1 additional projector for every 75 users	Additional projectors, the number based on program needs and availability of materials

Considerations in making choices:

1. Materials selected meet appropriate standards in projected-image quality in relation to size of intended audience.
2. Selection takes into consideration content areas—such as the sciences, physical education, and industrial education—in which this format offers potential strengths, e.g., short lengths, repeatability, and ease of use of cartridge-loaded films.
3. 8mm films produced by students and staff are incorporated in the collection on the basis of quality and need.
4. Both cartridge-loaded and open-reel films are considered for acquisition.
5. Consideration is given to standardization of Super 8mm formats used within a school and among schools sharing materials.
6. Selection of Super 8mm projectors reflects attention to the durability of the equipment which is subject to heavy use, including home circulation.
7. Both cartridge-loaded and open-reel projectors are considered for purchase.
8. The stop-motion (still frame) feature is a desirable option on Super 8mm projectors.
9. Provisions are made for rear screen projection of Super 8mm films, especially for use by small groups in media centers, laboratories, and shops.

BASE COLLECTION IN THE SCHOOL	EXTENDED PROVISIONS

AUDITORY FORMATS

AUDIO RECORDINGS: TAPES, CASSETTES, DISCS, AND AUDIO CARDS

1,500 to 2,000 items or 3 to 4 per user	Access to 5,000 items from the individual school's collection and loans from other sources

AUDIO EQUIPMENT: TAPE RECORDERS AND RECORD PLAYERS

30 audio reproduction units (open-reel and cassette tape recorders, stereo and monaural record players)	Highly individualized programs will require additional audio reproduction units, in the ratio of 1 per 5 users
Listening units: 1 set of earphones for each audio reproduction unit and 1 portable listening unit per 25 users	Access to specialized headsets to meet specific user needs may be provided from a district collection
Audio card units: available in sufficient quantity for use on a shared basis	Sufficient audio card units for permanent assignment to specific user locations

Considerations in making choices:

1. Auditory formats, offering content ranging from music to documentaries to drill materials, promote individualized development of listening skills and aural literacy.
2. Materials selected meet high standards in quality of audio reproduction, insuring intelligibility to the user.
3. Materials selected are evaluated for adequacy in fidelity, full frequency, and non-distortion of the original sound.
4. In choice of format(s), consideration is given to ease of use, availability of materials, and ability to produce recordings locally.
5. Blank tapes are provided for production of recordings by users and staff.
6. Equipment is selected carefully to insure accurate, high quality reproduction of the original sound.
7. Ease of equipment operation relative to intended use is considered in selection.

8. Equipment selection insures the provision of compatible units for use in synchronized audio productions.
9. Access to editing and mixing equipment is provided for users.
10. Open-reel and cassette tape duplicating equipment, needed for extensive collections of auditory materials, is provided at the district level and may be needed also in individual schools which make extensive use of auditory materials.

EDUCATIONAL BROADCAST RADIO

5 AM and FM receivers, plus a central distribution system

Access to specialized programs through public-service broadcasting and through special sources, e.g., university and state agencies

Considerations in making choices:

1. The media program identifies, obtains, and makes available to users program information, including guides and manuals when available from producers of educational broadcasting programs.
2. In districts that provide a broadcasting station access to sub-channel carriers for instructional purposes is considered.

TACTILE FORMATS

GAMES AND TOYS

400 to 750 items

Access to a sizeable district-level collection

Computer access from the district level may be provided for use with simulation games

Considerations in making choices:

1. Collections include materials chosen to augment the curriculum and to stimulate user interest.
2. Both commercially produced and locally developed games and toys are considered for inclusion in the collection.
3. Selection criteria emphasize a high degree of aesthetic appeal that invites handling of the objects in the process of use.

BASE COLLECTION IN THE SCHOOL	EXTENDED PROVISIONS

4. The collection includes materials for individual as well as group use.
5. Games and toys are repackaged as necessary to promote convenience, durability, and appeal in intended use.

MODELS AND SCULPTURE

200 to 500 items

Access to sizeable collections available from the school district and other agencies, including community resources

Considerations in making choices:

1. Models and sculpture reproductions exhibit a high degree of verisimilitude.
2. Items selected are sufficiently sturdy to withstand handling and examination by users.

SPECIMENS

200 to 400 items

Access to larger collections available from the school district and other agencies, including loan collections from zoos and museums

Considerations in making choices:

1. The collection makes adequate provision for specimens of long-term use, short-term use, and those which may be expendable.
2. Preserved specimens are selected with consideration for exactitude of representation and motivational appeal to the user.
3. Use of live specimens, where permitted, conforms with care to the rules and recommendations of humane societies.

INSTRUCTIONAL SYSTEMS, INCLUDING TEXTBOOKS

Types and quantities vary with program needs

81

Considerations in making choices:

1. Choices in instructional systems range from series of textbooks to multimedia packages of instructional materials to complex systems that combine materials and equipment in a program designed to meet precisely defined instructional objectives.
2. Emphasis is placed on the provision of a variety of instructional materials, including basic and supplementary texts and other instructional programs.
3. The organization, housing, distribution, and inventory of instructional systems, including textbooks, is recommended as a function of the school media program. This function requires the provision of one or more media aides, as needed, working with media professionals and teachers. In cases where instructional systems that include extensive hardware components are employed, a media technician may be needed to keep instructional equipment operating on a continuous basis. In addition, media center facilities will require adequate space for housing instructional systems.
4. Textbooks and other instructional programs may be assigned to individual classrooms or other locations within the school for extended periods of time. Instructional packages that include a variety of materials used by students, individually, as well as in classrooms, are housed in media centers for maximum accessibility (except as they may be assigned to classrooms for periods of time).
5. Media professionals participate with classroom teachers, curriculum consultants, and other staff in the selection of appropriate instructional systems.

MISCELLANEOUS EQUIPMENT

OPAQUE PROJECTORS

1 per media center
and
1 per 500 users (or 1 per floor in multistory building)

BASE COLLECTION IN THE SCHOOL	EXTENDED PROVISIONS

MICROPROJECTORS

1 per media center and 1 or more additional per school	Quantity sufficient to meet the needs of students and teachers in courses making extensive use of microprojectors

AUDITORIUM AND LARGE-GROUP PROJECTION EQUIPMENT

Auditorium-type 10″ x 10″ overhead projector

Screen with antikeystone device, and width equal to one-sixth the distance between the farthest viewer and the screen

16mm projector(s), auditorium-type, with high intensity light source

2″ x 2″ automatic slide projector, with high intensity light source

All projectors equipped with lenses matched to projection distance and screen size

PROJECTION CARTS

Ratio of projection carts to items of equipment is based on portability and distribution requirements, as well as storage space Cart height is appropriate to type of equipment and age of students	1 per motion picture, overhead, and opaque projector; video tape recorder; and classroom model tape recorder

PROJECTION SCREENS

1 permanently mounted screen per teaching station, usually 70″ x 70″ in size (a width of one-sixth the distance between the farthest viewer and the screen), with antikeystone provisions

BASE COLLECTION IN THE SCHOOL	EXTENDED PROVISIONS

Additional screens of suitable size, as needed, for individual and small group use; white matte walls can be used as projection surfaces

Multi-image projection requires larger or multiple screening surfaces

CLOSED-CIRCUIT TELEVISION

All new construction includes provisions for reception of closed-circuit television in the media center and in each teaching station

Older buildings are wired for closed-circuit television reception when television programming is initiated

A complete distribution system of at least six channels is available in a school so that broadcast TV 2500 MHZ, CATV, UHF, or VHF can be received; signals can be distributed to each teaching station from the central television reception area and/or a central studio; signals can be fed into the system from any teaching station; and signals are available simultaneously

LOCAL PRODUCTION EQUIPMENT: ADDITIONAL CONSIDERATIONS

Note: Basic requirements include the following items of equipment (in addition to other items listed in the foregoing categories).

Note: Other types of equipment needed vary with the school and district production programs. Types include (but may not be limited to) the following items.

Copying machines
1 per media center
and
1 per 500 users

Duplication machines
1 per media center
and
1 per 500 users

Press(es)

Dry mount press
1 per building, with platen-size approximately 18″ x 23″ and tacking iron

Rotary laminator

84

BASE COLLECTION IN THE SCHOOL	EXTENDED PROVISIONS

Paper cutters

    1 cutter (30″ or 36″) in media center
      and
    Additional cutters to meet user demands

Transparency makers   Diazo printer and developer

    1 thermal unit (unless included in copying machines, above)
    1 photocopier   Copy camera, 8″ x 10″
                              Equipped darkroom

Typewriters for graphics production   Mechanical lettering devices

    1 typewriter with large (10–12 point) size type and carbon ribbon. Variable spacing is optional.

Cameras and related equipment

    Cartridge-load slide-format camera with copy stand   35mm single-lens reflex camera
                              35mm half-frame camera with appropriate accessories
                              Large-format roll- or sheet-film camera, 2¼″ x 2¼″ or larger
    Super 8mm camera   16mm camera
    Light box   Programmer
                              Dissolve unit

Videotape equipment

    Videotape recorder, ½″ or ¾″   Switcher, video and audio
    Video camera(s)   Film chain

Film and video production equipment

    Film splicers, 16mm and Super 8mm   Film rewind
                                Film editors
                                Storyboard
                                Simple animation stand
                                Portable chalkboard

BASE COLLECTION IN THE SCHOOL	EXTENDED PROVISIONS

Audiotape production equipment

Tape splicers	Audiotape recorder with synchronizer
	Audiomixer, with monaural and stereo capacity

Considerations in making choices:

1. Types and amounts of local production equipment needed in the school reflect the scope and amount of media production performed within the school and the availability of production services at the district level.
2. Specialized equipment is selected on the basis of program needs and use requirements.
3. Selection of equipment takes into consideration the alternatives currently available, reflecting changes in technology.
4. School programs that emphasize filmmaking and photography require substantial increases in the collection of school-owned cameras and related equipment.

Facilities for media programs should support and enhance program activities, contributing to their efficiency of operation. The collection gains power with good facilities, equipment gets more use, production increases, and learners return readily to the media center. All users prefer surroundings that enable them to complete tasks in a satisfying way, whether they are staff members, teachers, or students.

GUIDING PRINCIPLES

1. The development of educational specifications for media program facilities is the responsibility of the director of the district media program, who works with media personnel, administrators, architects, and others concerned with the needed facilities.
2. The head of the school media program is responsible for evaluating facilities for the school media program and makes recommendations to the principal and the director of the district media program.
3. Planning involves representatives of all user groups, including media personnel, administrators, curriculum consultants, teachers, students, and community members. The group organized to develop educational specifications is small enough to operate effectively. Consultant assistance is obtained as needed from various specialists.
4. Planning for media program facilities is initiated as soon as the decision is made to construct, expand, or renovate school district or individual school facilities.

5. Planning takes into consideration the goals, characteristics, and other factors, including community and regional resources, that influence requirements for media program facilities.
6. Educational specifications for media program facilities are developed in written form.
7. Planning provides for media program facilities that are

appropriate to educational and media program goals and objectives

functional in design

attractive in appearance

located for maximum accessibility to users

designed for optimum functional relationships among areas within the media center, any satellite media centers, and the total school plant

flexible enough to permit adaptation to changing uses, to developing educational technology, and to other factors influencing media programs.

District Program Facilities

Facilities for the district media program are designed and provided on the basis of the number of schools and the size of the student population, as well as geographic characteristics, legal controls, and the district educational program and the media program's response to it. Factors to be considered in planning district media program facilities include the following questions:

Is the district located in a rural or urban area?

What effect do geographic factors have on the location of the district media center?

Is it feasible to contract with another district for some (or all) of the media services which need to be offered?

Does the district now have contractual arrangements with other districts for other types of services and do they relate to the media program?

Is the school district divided into administrative sub-units?

What financial factors in the district influence the scope and variety of district media program elements?

Is the present district administrative center located in one or several buildings? Is space currently available in any of these buildings? Will new construction be required?

The facilities for the district media program should be in the school district administrative center to provide maximum convenience in access, use, and communication. If the entire district program cannot be accommodated there, priority should be given to the media program administrative area, the professional materials collection, conference areas, and the media selection and evaluation center, in order to make these program elements accessible to curriculum specialists and committees, as well as to school personnel.

Plans for district media program facilities should take into consideration the following desirable characteristics:

Areas devoted to staff development programs are designed as models of effective teaching/learning spaces

Adequate parking is provided for all who will attend workshops, training sessions, demonstrations, and meetings

Facilities are available for use during after-school hours and during vacation periods

Functional and aesthetically pleasing furniture, equipment, and supplies are provided

Provision is made for equipment associated with production, evaluation, and use of materials

Adequate electrical outlets, light control, telephone and intercommunication devices, air conditioning, and sound control are provided as needed

Temperature and humidity controls are provided to prevent deterioration of collections.

Recommendations for district media program facilities follow.

AREAS	CONSIDERATIONS
Planning and Administration	Private office for the director and office areas for media professionals. Adjacent to curriculum specialists.
Consultative Service and Staff Development	Area for demonstration and staff development programs. Sound and light controls.
	Conference areas and meeting rooms, as needed. Portable walls to increase flexibility. Sound and light control. Area may be combined with media selection and evaluation center.
Film and Videotape Collections	Space for housing, rewinding, cleaning, and repair of film and videotape materials. Temperature and humidity controls. Located adjacent to shipping. Preview area.
Professional Library	Provides housing for all types of materials and associated equipment. Accommodates reading, study, listening, and viewing by users. Provides for circulation of materials to district staff and to schools.
	Area is accessible during, before, and after regular school hours and during vacation periods.
Media Selection and Evaluation Center	Accommodates all types of materials and associated equipment. Provides adequate space for individual and group viewing and listening without restricting access to or use of collection. Temperature, humidity, and light controls.
	May be part of professional library area; may be located adjacent to processing center.
Processing Center	Areas for receiving, cataloging, processing, and distribution. Space for office area, typists, processing clerks. Storage space for materials, supplies, and equipment. Space must allow for efficient work flow.
	Adequate electrical outlets, telephone and communication systems, sink(s), temperature and humidity control.

AREAS	CONSIDERATIONS
	Requires easy access from outside for shipping and receiving.
	Consider relationships to: media selection and evaluation center, production services, data processing, and business office.
Equipment Services: Evaluation, Maintenance, and Loan	Areas for inspection and repair of equipment. Storage areas for equipment (new items, loan items, and items scheduled for repair) and for parts and supplies.
Production Services:	Work area(s) for professional staff, technicians, and aides.
	Storage space for various sizes and dimensions of materials used and produced in the center.
	Space for packing and shipping materials produced in the center.
Graphics and Photography	Space for production of art work, with accompanying storage for work and supplies.
	Adequate paper storage space located near machines.
	Refrigeration equipment for photographic and diazo supplies.
	Air-conditioned darkroom with light locks and warning system.
Audiotape Production	Space for recorders and duplicators. Storage space for master tapes and duplicates.
	Soundproof room(s), as needed.
Radio Studio	Recording studio and control booth for live production with adequate sound control (*see* p. 102). May combine with or locate near production services area.

AREAS	CONSIDERATIONS
Television Production	Consider as alternatives for district television production: Contracting for television production, use of regional, state, or other programming, use of ministudios and portable videotape units.
	Area includes offices, studio(s), control room, and storage and work area. Adequate climate control for efficiency and comfort of operation. (See p. 103.)

School Program Facilities

Facilities for the school media program should be sufficient to underwrite its capabilities in serving the total program of the school of which it is a part. A spread of differences exists in goals and objectives and the characteristics of school populations. There are also variations between the requirements of elementary and secondary schools, and at all levels, instructional specializations call for alternatives in housing media program elements and relating functional areas.

Because good facilities are motivational and the lack of them actually depresses the fulfillment of program goals, they warrant special consideration before new schools are planned and existing schools are remodeled. For these reasons, the media program facilities should be reviewed regularly when evaluating the extent to which the school is achieving its objectives. Questions such as the following series should be asked when developing specifications, and the responses should be tabulated and carefully studied:

What is the student population to be served?
What is the anticipated maximum enrollment?
What are the significant characteristics of the students? Age levels? Special needs? Other?
What is the educational philosophy and the nature of the instructional program of the school?
Is instruction textbook-centered, teacher-oriented, or student-oriented? What emphasis is given to individualized instruction and independent study?

Is the school organized by grade level, department, schools within the school, self-contained class-rooms, or open-space areas?

Are there fixed class periods or modular scheduling?

Are mini-courses or other forms of short courses or alternative instructional programs offered?

Do students participate in designing learning experiences?

What effect does the design of the school have on the location of media facilities?

Is it a single level or multilevel building? A campus-type or multibuilding school?

Is all school audiovisual equipment stored in the media center or are decentralized storage areas used? What security arrangements are needed for equipment storage and distribution?

Should satellite media centers be planned in addition to the central media facility?

Where are the shipping, loading, elevator, and general storage facilities in the school?

Which of the following channels are provided in the school?

    Telephone and/or public address system(s)
    Closed-circuit television
    Dial access systems
    Broadcast radio and television

Is it anticipated that students and staff will use the media center singly; in small and large groups; in class-size groups; in combinations of these patterns, with what frequency for each?

Will the media center be used by community groups, night school classes or adult education classes?

Are there alternative or open school programs offered within the school concurrently with the regular program or on weekends, summers, evenings?

Which of the following types of production activities are provided by the school media program?

    Graphics production
    Printing

Photography
Super 8mm and/or 16mm film production
Television production
Audio production
What media services are offered to the school by the
district media program?
16mm film and videotape library
Professional library
Media selection and evaluation center
Acquisition, cataloging, and processing center
Maintenance and repair of equipment and
materials
Graphics and other production services?
Which?
Television and/or radio production
What media resources are available to the school or to
the district from community sources or from par-
ticipation by the school or the district in a net-
work?

Plans for the school media program facilities should take into
consideration the following desirable characteristics:

The school media center is located to provide easy
access and encourage frequent use.
The arrangement of facilities supports usage, with a
traffic flow that minimizes interruptions and distrac-
tions.
While facilities are primarily for the user, there are
adequate provisions for comfortable and efficient
working arrangements for the staff.
The facilities of the media center create an environment
that encourages the use of alternative media, that
sponsors inquiry, and that motivates every type of
student to use the collection and to draw upon media
program services.
Viewing, listening, and reading areas are properly
shielded from production and conference areas.
Facilities are available for use during and after school
hours and during vacation periods.

Provision is made for equipment associated with production, evaluation, and use of materials.
Adequate electrical outlets, light control, telephone and
intercommunication devices, air conditioning, and
sound control are provided as needed.
Temperature and humidity controls are provided to
prevent deterioration of collections.

As needed facilities are identified, decisions are reached concerning areas to be included and their size and relationships. Within the
media center and any accompanying satellite centers, all areas are
interrelated to promote the effective operation of the media program
and any given area may be planned to accommodate one or more
functions. Decisions concerning relationships among areas reflect
the needs of the individual school and determinations of area requirements are based on program activities.

The recommendations which follow are based on the needs of a
school with 1,000 (or fewer) students. These recommendations can
be adjusted to other populations, but all areas do not increase pro-
portionately; for example, the space for storing back issues of periodicals in a school of 4,000 students is not four times that of a
school of 1,000. Suggested square footage is supplied for each area,
but these figures should not be totaled as the basis for overall area
recommendations.

AREAS	RELATIONSHIPS AND SPECIAL CONSIDERATIONS	SUGGESTED SPACE ALLOCATIONS
Circulation (for display, exhibits, copy-ing equipment, card catalogs, periodical indexes, charging)	RELATIONSHIPS. Near main en-trance; near reserve collection; near work area; near equipment storage area	800 sq. ft.
	SPECIAL CONSIDERATIONS. Should copying equipment be placed here, elsewhere, or in several locations? Media centers with more than one floor or multiple major entrances require space allocations at each	200 sq. ft. additional for circulation area in each satellite center

95

AREAS	RELATIONSHIPS AND SPECIAL CONSIDERATIONS	SUGGESTED SPACE ALLOCATIONS
	entrance. Satellite centers need to provide for these areas. Periodical indexes should be adjacent to periodical storage, current periodicals, and the microform periodical collection. Card (or other) catalogs should be near reference collection or general reference area. Satellite centers require space for catalogs.	
Reading, Browsing, Listening, Viewing	RELATIONSHIPS. Reference area near card catalog, periodical indexes. Magazines near periodical indexes, microform readers.	15 to 30 percent of enrollment at 40 sq. ft. per student
	SPECIAL CONSIDERATIONS. Some instructional programs may require ⅓ to ¾ of the student body to be in the media center or satellite centers at any one time. No more than 100 students should be seated in any one area. In elementary schools, a storytelling area should be located away from noisy areas. At least 30 percent of the seating capacity should provide for individual listening and viewing. The area should be ducted and wired for power and coaxial cable distribution. Modular floor outlets should be considered. Rows of carrels and other institutional seating arrangements should be avoided. Where carrels are used they should be equipped with listening and viewing capability. In areas planned specifically for listening and view-	A minimum of 9 sq. ft. of floor space is required per single carrel. Some carrels may take 15 sq. ft.

AREAS	RELATIONSHIPS AND SPECIAL CONSIDERATIONS	SUGGESTED SPACE ALLOCATIONS
	ing avoid the possibility of conflicting audio messages and/or visual distraction. Mix seating types of chairs and tables; include lounge-type seating.	
Open Access Materials Housing (Usually integrated into reading, browsing, listening, and viewing areas)	RELATIONSHIPS. Various media formats may be housed on separate shelves or in storage cabinets or interfiled on open shelves according to subject. Reserve area may be open or closed and should be near the circulation area. SPECIAL CONSIDERATIONS. Shelving and materials housing in elementary schools is of a style and height appropriate for the age group. Type(s) and amount of open access materials housing depend on whether intershelving of formats is planned, or whether materials will be housed by format. Accommodation for all types of formats, including kits, games, and realia, is planned.	Shelving and/or cabinets to accommodate a minimum of 40 items per student, exclusive of textbooks
Small Group Listening and Viewing	RELATIONSHIPS. Small group listening and viewing may be accommodated in open areas of the media center via use of headsets, rear-screen projection, etc. Additional small group listening and viewing areas may be necessary. SPECIAL CONSIDERATIONS. Space provided for listening and viewing areas is in addition to space allocated for conference rooms (which	Minimum of 150 sq. ft. per area

97

AREAS	RELATIONSHIPS AND SPECIAL CONSIDERATIONS	SUGGESTED SPACE ALLOCATIONS
	should be equipped also to accommodate this function). The area(s) should have electrical and TV inputs and outlets, permanent wall screen, and acoustical treatment.	
Conference Areas	RELATIONSHIPS. Locate in quiet area of media center. Consider housing here special collections of materials for which continuous access is not required.	Minimum of 3 conference rooms of 150 sq. ft. each
	SPECIAL CONSIDERATIONS. Greater flexibility is achieved when some conference areas are adjoining, and movable walls may be used to combine or divide a series of areas. Sound control is necessary as is provision for light control. Areas should be equipped with electrical and TV inputs and outlets. These areas may be used for typing as needed and as areas for temporary display or highlighting of special collections.	
Group Projects and Instruction	RELATIONSHIPS. Adjacent to reference and open materials housing, and to catalogs and indexes, if possible.	900–1200 sq. ft.
	SPECIAL CONSIDERATIONS. Flexible space, at least classroom size, equipped for audio and visual presentations. Consider housing special collections of materials here. Consider providing storage for student projects in process.	

AREAS	RELATIONSHIPS AND SPECIAL CONSIDERATIONS	SUGGESTED SPACE ALLOCATIONS
Administration	RELATIONSHIPS. Office for head of the media program should be near the professional collection and easily accessible from rest of school.	
	SPECIAL CONSIDERATIONS. Desk space for media personnel should be provided in appropriate areas of the media center. In addition, the media professionals should have office space for program planning and related work. Arrangement and location of office areas depends upon the total configuration of the media center and its internal organization.	Desk space for media staff as necessary; 150 sq. ft. per media professional
Work Space	RELATIONSHIPS. Locate near production and distribution facilities and equipment storage, when possible. Needs access to corridor and to elevator or loading dock.	300–400 sq. ft.
	SPECIAL CONSIDERATIONS. Total amount of work space may be provided in one area, in smaller schools; large schools may need several work areas. Provision for shelving and storage of supplies. Requires sinks, running water, electrical outlets. Increase amount of space if cataloging and processing are performed in the school.	
Equipment Storage and Distribution	RELATIONSHIPS. Locate near corridor and freight elevator. Consider location in relation to production area and staff work space.	Minimum of 400 sq. ft.

AREAS	RELATIONSHIPS AND SPECIAL CONSIDERATIONS	SUGGESTED SPACE ALLOCATIONS
	SPECIAL CONSIDERATIONS. Provide for availability of equipment in the production and listening/viewing areas of the media center. Plan necessary provisions for security of equipment. Large schools or those with characteristics making distribution difficult will need to provide for decentralized equipment storage and distribution.	
Maintenance and Repair	RELATIONSHIPS. Near freight elevator, loading dock; adjacent to equipment storage and distribution area. SPECIAL CONSIDERATIONS. Area may be combined with equipment storage and distribution area. Additional space is required if major maintenance and repair is performed within the school.	120–200 sq. ft.
Media Production Laboratory	RELATIONSHIPS. Consider locating adjacent to equipment storage and distribution area. SPECIAL CONSIDERATIONS. Provide housing for equipment and materials used in production, and shelving and storage for supplies. Requires temperature and humidity controls, refrigeration, sinks, running water, electrical outlets, and counter space. Sound control is needed for audio production. Plan space arrangements in terms of production methods used and work flow.	Minimum of 800 sq. ft. Additional space in schools in which students produce materials

AREAS	RELATIONSHIPS AND SPECIAL CONSIDERATIONS	SUGGESTED SPACE ALLOCATIONS
Darkroom	RELATIONSHIPS. The darkroom area, if included in the media center, should be adjacent to the media production laboratory. (A darkroom may be provided elsewhere in the school.)	150–200 sq. ft.
	SPECIAL CONSIDERATIONS. Requires sinks, running water, electrical outlets, light locks, refrigeration, counter space, adequate ventilation.	
Professional Collection for Faculty	RELATIONSHIPS. Consider in relation to location of teacher's lounge, media production laboratory, department offices, main media center.	Minimum of 600 sq. ft.
	SPECIAL CONSIDERATIONS. May plan for use as faculty group meeting or conference area. Provide for listening and viewing and for selection and evaluation of new materials and equipment. Emphasize lounge atmosphere.	
Stacks	RELATIONSHIPS. Locate near reserve area, if appropriate. Consider location in relation to periodical storage.	Minimum of 400 sq. ft.
	SPECIAL CONSIDERATIONS. Adequate lighting. Provide for tables and seating as necessary, depending on types of materials stored in stacks. Include additional stack space as needed to store textbooks.	Additional space for textbook storage

101

AREAS	RELATIONSHIPS AND SPECIAL CONSIDERATIONS	SUGGESTED SPACE ALLOCATIONS
Magazine and Newspaper Storage	RELATIONSHIPS. Locate near periodical indexes, current periodical shelving, and microform readers. SPECIAL CONSIDERATIONS. Consider space needed for microform readers and reader-printers. Consider installation of copying equipment in this area.	Minimum of 400 sq. ft.

Additional media program facilities as determined by school needs follow.

Computerized Learning Laboratory	RELATIONSHIPS. Adjacent to group project and instruction area. SPECIAL CONSIDERATIONS. Constitutes an area within the media center complex. Should have response capability.	Depends on nature of computer usage
Storage and Control for Remote Access		Depends on nature of remote access system
Radio Studio	RELATIONSHIPS. May be located near television production area (if any). SPECIAL CONSIDERATIONS. If radio studio is provided, classroom facilities may be needed. This function may be provided instead at district level.	500 sq. ft. (20' x 25') with additional space for control

AREAS	RELATIONSHIPS AND SPECIAL CONSIDERATIONS	SUGGESTED SPACE ALLOCATIONS
Television Studio	RELATIONSHIPS. Should be convenient to media production area. SPECIAL CONSIDERATIONS. Area must be soundproof. Classroom facilities may be needed. Studio capability may be provided instead at district level. Consider as alternatives for school television production: ministudios and portable videotape units.	1600 sq. ft. studio (40′ x 40′); additional control space; 15′ ceilings, 14′ x 12′ doors
Television Storage	RELATIONSHIPS. Adjacent to television studio. SPECIAL CONSIDERATIONS. May need to consider relation to other shipping and storage facilities if TV props and visuals are shared between schools.	Minimum of 800 sq. ft.
Television Office	RELATIONSHIPS. Adjacent to television studio and storage areas.	150 sq. ft.

EQUIPMENT AND FURNITURE FOR SCHOOL MEDIA CENTERS

MATERIALS HOUSING. In selecting shelving and other storage units for the materials collection, types and quantities depend on such factors as types of formats represented, how materials are housed —intershelved or by format—and the anticipated size of collection. (*See* chapter 6, Collections.)

EQUIPMENT HOUSING. Shelving, storage units, and floor space accommodate the equipment in the collection. Types and amounts of housing should support maximum use and vary with such factors as assignment of equipment to specified locations and the anticipated size of the collection. (*See* chapter 6, Collections.)

FURNITURE. Furniture in the media center is functional, aesthetically pleasing, and consonant with the tastes of the users. In establishing specifications, it should be remembered that of itself furniture creates an environment which can set moods that lead to or inhibit inquiry and user fulfillment.

Height of furniture students use and shelving and storage units accessible to them is determined by the ages of the pupil population. Types of furniture include the following:

> *Chairs*: study chairs; easy or lounge chairs; cushions, hassocks, or benches; stacking chairs are useful in multipurpose areas
>
> *Tables*: sturdy tables for individuals and 2–4 students; informal, lounge-area tables; reference and periodical index tables; project tables for production and work areas; conference tables; typing tables; counters needed in work areas
>
> *Carrels*: with and without listening and viewing capabilities
>
> *Desks and chairs*: for media personnel, includes work stools for counter-height work stations
>
> *Specialized furniture*: circulation desk; book-return drop or bin; atlas and dictionary stands; vertical files, both legal and letter size; storage cabinets with locks for supplies and equipment; display shelves, cases, cabinets; bulletin boards.

Media Programs: District and School focuses on the user of media programs. The central concern is the quality of the educational experience for the learner. Quality district and school media programs undergird and extend educational opportunities by providing the resources for teaching and learning: for working directly with students in the development of print, aural, and visual literacies, for providing the skills of learning how to learn, self-directed learning, and the means of creative expression and communication; for working with teachers in design and implementation of curriculum and the effective utilization of media; for participating with administrators and consultants in the complex tasks of program development and administration; and for extending opportunities for all users of media programs through utilization of resources and services available from the community, regional programs, state agencies, and networks.

This publication anticipates the move toward greater diversity in educational strategies in order to reach the many needs of the specific publics served. It suggests ways and means that encourage the development of a media program tailored to the individual educational program, district or school, of which it is a part. It recognizes that educational programs and media programs develop together to promote the intellectual, physical, emotional, aesthetic, and spiritual growth of users.

Similarly, the document recognizes the interdependence between district and school media programs, the responsibilities of the state education agency, the imperative for cooperation with related community agencies, and the opportunities afforded by regional media programs and by networks.

The American Association of School Librarians and the Association for Educational Communications and Technology recognize that

105

the kinds of relationships between and among media personnel, learners, teachers, administrators and consultants, and community members reflect the quality of the media program as each user interacts with the media, media processes, and environments provided. Both associations strongly support media programs that expand rather than curtail individual options, that recognize the necessity for individual and program objectives, and that nurture warm, satisfying human experiences.

Media Programs: District and School recognizes options and supports intelligent selection from educational alternatives on the basis of rational, empirically based approaches to the solution of educational problems. Selection and provision of appropriate program components requires that media professionals be sensitive to the changing nature of society, be able to work intelligently and creatively, and be able to employ a wide range of alternatives. In the decade ahead, no area of the school program has more potential to improve learning than does the media program, as it responds to the increasing potential offered by systems of communication. At every level—national, state, regional, district, and school—media professionals must consider the implications of increased technological applications to the improvement of education. In keeping with these considerations, this publication enumerates general principles to be applied to media program operations, suggests points to be considered before programming decisions are made and offers ranges in quantitative provisions for media programs based on options in district and school media programs and resources available from other levels. The key to program development is flexibility based on purpose and effectiveness.

Both sponsoring associations recognize the need for a spread of competencies in media program staffing. Only through differentiated staffing patterns can individual and collective expertise be assembled to plan, implement, and evaluate comprehensive media programs.

A basic assumption made throughout this document is that the quality of contact users have with materials, machines, personnel, and environments determines the quality of the media program. Lists of desirable and observable user activities are provided to illustrate what users may be found doing in quality media programs. These lists describe activities that are initiated, implemented, and fulfilled through the management of program components. In this sense the potential of the media program, district or school, relates to its effectiveness in establishing relationships that enable users to meet personal and program goals.

In *Media Programs: District and School*, AASL and AECT call for media programs that are user-centered, that promote flexibility in practice based on intelligent selection from many alternatives, and that are derived from well-articulated learning and program objectives. The purpose of these guidelines is to expand the possibilities for media program planners and to provide a tool for broadening concepts of the potential that media programs offer for improving the educational experience. Now the challenge is made to all media professionals to use the document in their own ways to increase educational opportunities at all levels through the design and implementation of effective, responsive media programs.

The meaning of terms varies in practice and even in parts of the country. Words and phrases are also subject to change as new developments occur in the fields they describe. A list of terms with accompanying amplification is provided to clarify usage within this book; it is not intended to establish standard definitions, even though it will undoubtedly verify or extend assumed meanings.

Media Personnel

Media personnel are persons with specialized interest and training who develop and carry out media programs as an integral part of the curriculum. They include all the professional and support members of a media staff.

Media Professional. Any media person, certificated or not, who qualifies by training and position to make professional judgments and to delineate and maintain media programs or program components. Media professionals may include media specialists, television or film producers, instructional developers, radio station managers, and technical processing (cataloging) specialists, whose duties and responsibilities are professional in nature

Media Specialist. A person with appropriate certification and broad professional preparation, both in education and media, with competencies to carry out a media program. The media specialist is the basic media professional in the school program

Director of District Media Program. A media professional with appropriate certification and advanced managerial, administrative, and supervisory competencies who qualifies for an administrative or supervisory position

Head of School Media Program. A media specialist with managerial competencies who is designated as responsible for the media program at the individual school level. Qualifications vary with such factors as the size of the school, size of media staff, and type of program

Media Technician. A member of the media staff with technical skills in such specialized areas as graphics production and display, information and materials processing, photographic production, operation and maintenance of audiovisual equipment, operation and maintenance of television equipment, and installation of systems components

Media Aide. A member of the media staff who performs clerical and secretarial tasks and assists as needed in the acquisition, maintenance, inventory, production, distribution, and utilization of materials and equipment

Media Support Personnel. All persons including technicians and aides who utilize specific skills and abilities to carry out program activities as delineated by professional staff members

Program

The media program is the total expression of all media functions including their delineation, their implementation in working with users, and their evaluation and projection. It is realized through interaction among personnel, processes, and information sources. *Process* is the specialized adaptation of scientific procedures applied to achieving a specific task or an established goal. *Information* is the communication or reception of knowledge and *media* are all of the forms and channels used in the transmittal process. The point at which an information transfer or exchange occurs is an *interface*. The media program, therefore, can be described as patterns of interfacings among program components, e.g., people, materials, machines, facilities, and environments managed by media professionals who establish and maintain relationships between or among the components.

School. An organized group of learners under a professional and administrative staff traditionally housed in a building or adjacent buildings, usually part of a larger operational unit

School Media Program. The media program for a school, conducted through an administrative subunit

School Media Center. An area or system of areas in the school where a full range of information sources, associated equipment, and services from media staff are accessible to students, school personnel, and the school community

District. A local basic administrative unit existing primarily to operate schools, public or nonpublic, or to contract for school services. A district may or may not be coterminous with the county, city, or town boundaries and may be identified by such terms as school system, basic administrative unit, local school system, or local educational agency

District Media Program. The media program that is conducted at the school district level through an administrative subunit

Region. A cooperative or legislated combination of districts

Regional Media Program. The media program conducted by a region

Process

Process, as used in this book, relates to a series of planned and related activities that lead to a particular result. District and school media programs use scientific processes that can be applied to a variety of educational problems. These processes include

Generating goals from educational purposes
Translating goals into objectives suitable for analysis

111

Analyzing objectives

Identifying constraints (physical, financial, time, legal, and policy factors)

Identifying variables (performance, time, policy, risk factors)

Generating alternatives

Conducting trade-off studies and selecting among alternatives

Developing prototypes

Conducting developmental testing programs

Administering field tests

Installing instructional systems

Designing monitoring systems.

The order and the comparative emphasis vary in accordance with the tasks.

This publication recognizes the necessity and value of applying scientific principles to educational activity. It further identifies media processes as basic avenues for achieving solutions to individual learning problems. Terms relating to the total educational program with special application to media processes are thus defined:

Educational Technology. The broad application of scientific processes to the solution of educational problems and the fulfillment of learners

Instructional Technology. That part of educational technology concerned with applying scientific processes to learning experiences

Instructional Design. The formulation and selection of management systems for instructional development

Instructional Systems Components. All resources which can be designed, utilized, and combined in a systematic manner with the intent of achieving learning

Instructional System(s). An integrated group of program components organized to accomplish stated objectives

112

Instructional Development. The solution of instructional problems through the design and application of instructional systems and their components

Instructional Product Design. The process of identifying or creating the most effective materials to meet the specific objectives of learning experiences

Members of Task Force I	Representing
ELSIE L. BRUMBACK Assistant Director, Field Services Division of Educational Media North Carolina State Department of Public Instruction Raleigh, NC	AECT
RUTH A. DAVIES Coordinator of Library Service North Hills School District Pittsburgh, PA	AASL
MILDRED P. FRARY Director, Library Services Instructional Materials Center Los Angeles Unified School District Los Angeles, CA	AASL
WILLIAM R. FULTON Professor of Education University of Oklahoma Norman, OK	AECT
RICHARD W. GILKEY Director, Educational Media Department Portland Public Schools Portland, OR	AECT
DAVID V. GUERIN Coordinator of Instructional Materials Garden City High School Garden City, NY	AECT

WILLIAM E. HUG   AASL
Associate Professor of Education
Teachers College
Columbia University
New York, NY

ROBERT F. JARECKE   AECT
Professor of Education and Director, Center for
    Instructional Media
California State University, Sacramento
Sacramento, CA

LEONE H. LAKE   AECT
Media Specialist/Teacher
South Beach Elementary School
Dade County Board of Public Instruction
Miami Beach, FL

PRISCILLA L. MOULTON   AASL
Director of Libraries
Public Schools of Brookline
Brookline, MA

ELIZABETH M. STEPHENS   AASL
Director, Library Resources
Pinellas County Public Schools
Clearwater, FL

CHRISTINA CARR YOUNG   AASL
Formerly Educational Specialist, ESEA Title II
Department of Library Science
District of Columbia Public Schools
Washington, DC

Members of Task Force II   Representing

LILLIAN L. BATCHELOR   AASL
Assistant Director in Charge, Libraries
School District of Philadelphia
Philadelphia, PA

JAMES W. CARRUTH   AECT
Director, Division of Educational Media
North Carolina State Department of Public
    Instruction
Raleigh, NC

115

ABRAHAM J. COHEN   AECT
Supervisor of Instructional Materials
  and School Libraries
White Plains Public Schools
White Plains, NY

THOMAS E. COLLINS   AECT
Media Supervisor
Division of Media Field Services
Department of Educational Media and Technology
Montgomery County Public Schools
Rockville, MD

WINIFRED E. DUNCAN   AASL
Supervisor, Division of Libraries
City of Chicago Board of Education
Chicago, IL

ELIZABETH T. FAST   AASL
Director of Media Services
Groton Public Schools
Groton, CT

BERNARD FRANCKOWIAK   AASL
School Library Supervisor
Wisconsin State Department of Public Instruction
Madison, WI

FRANZ FREDERICK   AECT
Assistant Professor, Media Sciences
Department of Education
Purdue University
West Lafayette, IN

JOSEPH F. GIORGIO   AECT
Coordinator, Learning Resources
Fairfield Public Schools
Fairfield, CT

WILLIAM F. GRADY   AECT
Chairman, Division of Educational Communications
Temple University
Philadelphia, PA

JANE A. HANNIGAN   AASL
Associate Professor
School of Library Service
Columbia University
New York, NY

BETTIE R. HELSER   AASL
Media Specialist
Unified School District 501
Topeka, KS

ARTHUR W. LALIME   AECT
Director, Instructional Materials Services
Darien Public Schools
Darien, CT

F. JOSEPH LAMPING   AECT
Coordinator, Resource Services Branch
Cincinnati Public Schools
Cincinnati, OH

ELIZABETH B. MANN   AASL
Associate Director of Learning Resources
Florida Mental Health Institute
Tampa, FL

JAMES M. MEAGHER   AECT
Director, Department of Educational Media
Penfield Central School
Penfield, NY

RUTH A. MOLINE   AASL
Director, Instructional Media Center
Educational Service Unit No. 2
Fremont, NE

JOHNNY M. SHAVER   AECT
Chief Consultant, Production and Technical Services
Division of Educational Media
North Carolina State Department of
    Public Instruction
Raleigh, NC

CLARK P. SHELBY   AECT
Administrative Assistant
Alhambra School District
Phoenix, AR

MARY ANN SWANSON   AASL
Supervisor of Media Services
Evanston Township High School
Evanston, IL

ROBERTA E. YOUNG   AASL
Formerly Director, Library Development
Office of Library Services
Colorado State Department of Education

ELINOR YUNGMEYER   AASL
Coordinator, Instructional Media
Oak Park Elementary Schools, District No. 97
Oak Park, IL

Members of Joint Editorial Revision Committee

TERESA J. DOHERTY
Supervisor, Instructional Media
Department of Educational Media and Technology
Montgomery County Public Schools
Rockville, MD

LEILA ANN DOYLE
Coordinator of Learning Resource Center
Indiana Vocational Technical College
Gary, IN

ELIZABETH T. FAST
Director of Media Services
Groton Public Schools
Groton, CT

RICHARD W. GILKEY
Director, Educational Media Department
Portland Public Schools
Portland, OR

MAE GRAHAM
Formerly Assistant Director
Division of Library Development and Services
Maryland State Department of Education

JANE A. HANNIGAN
Associate Professor
School of Library Service
Columbia University
New York, NY

ROBERT HEINICH
Professor of Education
Audiovisual Center
Indiana University
Bloomington, IN

WILLIAM E. HUG
Associate Professor
Teachers College
Columbia University
New York, NY

MARY FRANCES K. JOHNSON
Associate Professor
School of Education
University of North Carolina at Greensboro
Greensboro, NC

NINA N. MARTIN
Associate Professor
Graduate School of Library Service
University of Alabama
University, AL

JOHNNY M. SHAVER
Chief Consultant, Production and Technical Services
Division of Educational Media
North Carolina State Department of
    Public Instruction
Raleigh, NC

MARY W. TRAVILLIAN
Director, Area Six Resource Center
Marshalltown, IA

CAROLYN I. WHITENACK
Professor of Education and
Chairman, Media Sciences
Purdue University
West Lafayette, IN

ELINOR YUNGMEYER
Coordinator, Instructional Media
Oak Park Elementary Schools, District No. 97
Oak Park, IL

Ex-Officio Representatives

	Capacity
JOHN E. DOME Director, Instructional Resources Planning Miami University Oxford, OH	AECT Program Standards Committee Chairman
BERNARD FRANCKOWIAK School Library Supervisor Wisconsin State Department of Public Instruction Madison, WI	AASL President, 1973–74
FRANCES HATFIELD Coordinator of Instructional Materials Broward County School Board Fort Lauderdale, FL	AASL President, 1971–72
ROBERT HEINICH Professor of Education Audiovisual Center Indiana University Bloomington, IN	AECT President, 1970–71
HOWARD B. HITCHENS Executive Director Association for Educational Communications and Technology Washington, DC	
ROBERT F. JARECKE Professor of Education and Director, Center for Instructional Media California State University, Sacramento Sacramento, CA	AECT President, 1973–74

JERROLD E. KEMP
Coordinator, Instructional Development Services
Instructional Resources Center
San Jose State University
San Jose, CA

AECT President,
1972–73

RICHARD G. NIBECK
Deputy Executive Director
Association for Educational Communications
   and Technology
Washington, DC

P. E. PATTERSON
Consultant, Audiovisual Education
Bureau of Audiovisual and School Library
   Education
California State Department of Education
Sacramento, CA

AECT Liaison,
Task Force I

ELNORA M. PORTTEUS
Directing Supervisor, School Libraries
Cleveland Public Schools
Cleveland, OH

AASL President,
1972–73

ROWENA S. SADLER
Formerly Assistant Executive Secretary
American Association of School Librarians
Washington, DC

LU OUIDA VINSON
Executive Secretary
American Association of School Librarians
Chicago, IL

ROBERTA E. YOUNG
Formerly Director
Library Development
Office of Library Services
Colorado State Department of Education

AASL President,
1970–71

Academic preparation of media staff, 22, 23
Access and delivery systems, 9, 16, 19, 48; for district media program, 49, 52; for school media program, 52–53
Accountability techniques, 11
Accounting services, centralized, 49
Administration, 27; facilities for, 90, 99; of funds, 18; of state media program, 17. *See also* District media director; Head of school media program
Administration function of media program, 9
Advisory services, 16, 32
Aide, *see* Media aide
Audiomixer, 87
Audiotapes, 25, 79–80, 86; duplication, 30; production, 30, 46, 47, 91
Audiovisual materials, *see* Materials; individual names
Auditorium projection equipment, 83
Auditory materials, 79–80

Base collection for school media program, 68–86
Bibliographic service, providing, 8
Board of education and media programs, 16–17, 57
Books, school collection, 70
Browsing area, 96
Budget: administration, 27; allocations, 40, 60; criteria, 14; developing, 7, 8, 11, 12, 14, 27, 38–40, 60; for equipment and supplies, 47–48, 55; presentation, 40; requests, 32; for school media collection, 68

Cameras, 85
Carrels, 104

Cassettes, 79–80
Catalogers, 28
Cataloging, 52
Certification requirements for media staff, 19
Chairs for media center, 104
Circulation, 25, 53; area, 18, 95–96
Closed-circuit television, 84
Collections: components of, 63; developing, 9; development, cooperative approaches in, 63–64; district, 11, 18, 62, 64–65, 66–67; facilities for, 90; film, 28, 66, 76–78; funding for, 38–42; guiding principles for, 62–65; items per student, 69, 70; organization and arrangement, 63; reevaluation, 63, 65; of regional media program, 16; school, 14, 62, 63, 68–86; selection, 11, 62, 64–67; selection and evaluation center, 67; special, of regional program, 16; videotape, 28
Communication arts, 5
Communication skills, developing students' competence in, 8
Communication technology, 10
Computerized instruction, 16
Computerized learning laboratory, 102
Conference areas, 98
Consultative services, 16, 18; of district media program, 27; facilities for, 90
Contractual arrangements between school districts, 26
Cooperation among school districts, 25–26
Copying machines, 84
Cost-effectiveness principles, 48
Council of Chief State School Officers, 18
Creative expression, 14

Curriculum: design, 6–7, 10, 13, 31; development and implementation, 7; planning, 26, 31; program activities responding to goals, 14; and school media program, 15

Darkroom, 17, 85, 101
Data bases, 19
Decision-making: criteria for, 7; instructional, 21
Delivery systems, 48–49, 52–53
Design: curriculum, 6–7, 10, 13, 31; instructional, 37, 60, 112; of materials, 5, 46
Design function of media program, 6–7
Desks, 104
Diazo printer and developer, 85
Discs, audio, 79
Displays, 46
District media director, 12, 21, 25, 31; definition, 109–10; and purchasing, 42–43; responsibilities, 15, 26–27, 38, 39, 40, 56, 57, 87
District media program, 21; access and delivery systems, 49, 52; consultative service, 27; definition, 111; evaluation, 12, 59; facilities for, 88–92; planning and administration, 11, 27, 90–92; production of materials, 45–46; public information program, 57–58; requirements, variations in, 12–13; responsibilities of, 10–13; services offered to schools, 62, 94; staff, 21, 25–30, 55
Districts: annual expenditure per student, 40–42; collections, 11, 64–65, 66–67; cooperation among, and staffing, 25–26; definition of, 111; supplements to school collections, 62
Dry mount press, 84
Duplication machines, 84

ERIC, see Educational Resources Information Center
Educational radio, 16, 80
Educational Resources Information Center, 20
Educational technology, 112
Educational television, 16

Equipment: audio, 79–80; audiotape production, 86; circulation from media center, 53; evaluation, 63; examination, 65–67; film, 76–78, 85; filmstrip, 73; instructional, operation and use of, 24; locating, 25; maintenance, 24, 28–29, 54–55, 91, 100; microform, 72; production, 84–86; purchasing, 42, 43–44; selection, 32; services, 28–29, 91; slide, 74; storage and distribution, 99, 103–4; transparency, 74; video playback, 77; videotape, 85
Evaluation: of district media program, 12, 59; of equipment, 63; external, 59; of materials, 18, 63, 65–67; of media, 28, 63, 65, 90; of media programs, 7, 58–61; of media staff, 32; of school media program, 15, 60–61
Examination of materials and equipment, 65–67

Facilities for media programs, 87–104; new, developing educational specifications for, 9; school and district, designing, 11
Film collections: administration of, 28; district, 66; facilities for, 90; school, 76–78
Films: collections, see Film collections; producing, 24, 94; production equipment, 85; silent, 77–78; 16mm, 76–77; sound, 76–78; Super 8mm, 76–78
Filmstrips: equipment, 73; school collection, 73
Funding, 38–42, 68
Funds: administration of, 18
Furniture in media center, 104

Games, 80–81
Globes, school collection, 75
Graphics, 24; facilities for producing, 91–92; production, 24, 29, 45, 47, 91, 93; production, typewriter for, 85; school collection, 75
Group projects and instruction, area for, 98

Head of school media program, 13, 21, 26; definition, 110; office for,

99; responsibilities, 15, 31–32, 38, 53, 55, 58, 87

Information: access to, 19, 48–49, 52–53; definition, 110; organizing and indexing, 8; public, 9, 11, 14, 27, 32, 55–58; retrieval, 5; sources, 48; translating from one presentation form to another, 8
Information function of media program, 6, 8–9
In-service education, 14, 27, 32, 90; designing, 7
Instructional design, 37, 60, 112
Instructional development, 113
Instructional materials: design, 113; determining effectiveness, 7; regional collections of, 16
Instructional resources consultant, 7
Instructional sequences: determining effectiveness, 7; utilizing, 5
Instructional systems, 81–82; components, 112
Instructional technology, 112
Intellectual freedom, 6, 64–65
Interest fulfillment, 14
Interface, definition of, 110

Kits, designing, 46

Laboratory: computerized learning, 102; media production, 100
Laminator, rotary, 84
Leadership development programs, 18
Learning, creating alternative modes, 13
Legislative action for media program development, 17
Library, professional, 10, 14, 28, 90, 101; for district, 66–67
Library of Congress, 20
Library technical assistants, 28
Light box, 85
Listening: area, 96–98; developing competencies in, 8

Machine-Readable Cataloging program (MARC), 20
Magazines: school collection, 71; storage, 102
Maintenance of materials and equipment, 9, 11, 24, 28–29, 54–55, 91, 100
Maps, school collection, 75
Materials: access and delivery systems, 9, 16, 48–49, 52–53; assistance in use, 6, 8, 25; collections, see Collections; designing, 5; evaluation, 18, 63, 65–67; examination, 65–67; instructional, 7, 16, 113; instructional resources consultant, 7; locating and retrieving, 5, 25; maintenance, 9, 54–55, 100; open access, 97; processing, 24, 26, 28, 90–91; processing services, 48, 49; production, 1, 5, 6, 9, 11, 14, 24, 25, 29–30, 44–48, 84–86, 100–101; purchasing, 42, 43; selection, 11, 28, 32, 62, 64–65, 70–82, 86, 90; for self-instruction, developing, 7; for specific objectives, 5; storage, 103
Materials specialist, 7
Media: applications for specific purposes, recommending, 7; definition, 110; evaluation, 28, 63, 65, 90; utilization and curriculum design, 10. See also Materials; individual names
Media aide, 28, 33, 35; competencies of, 24; definition, 110; duties of, 24–25
Media center: instruction in use of, 8; operating, 14; school, 14, 93–103, 111
Media education, planning for, 19
Media personnel, see Media staff
Media professional, see Professional staff
Media program: activities of users in, 5–6, 60–61, 106–7; administration function, 9; components of, 4; concern for intellectual freedom, 6; consultation function, 6, 7–8; criteria for decision-making, 7; definition, 110–11; design function, 6–7; designing facilities, 11; development, 106; effective, developing, 37; evaluation, 7, 58–61; facilities, 9, 11, 87–104; information function, 6, 8–9; planning, 7, 11, 18, 27, 36–38; policies, 6; priorities, identifying, 7; public information, 9, 11, (Continued)

Media Programs (*Cont.*)
14, 27, 32, 55–58; purposes of, 4, 7, 21; resources, 4; staff, *see* Media staff; in state department of education, 17–19; value of, 5. *See also* District media program; School media program
Media selection and evaluation center, 67, 90
Media specialist: academic preparation, 22–23; competencies of, 22–23; definition, 109; proportion of to number of students, 33–34
Media staff, 5, 20–21, 22–26, 106; certification requirements, 19; and curriculum design, 6–7; development programs for, 14, 16, 27, 32, 90; district, 21, 25–30, 55; evaluation, 32; goals of, 4; for graphics production, 29; guiding principles for, 21; physical facilities for, 99; position classifications, 27; for printing services, 29; professional, *see* Professional staff; for school media program, 21, 30–35; selection, 11, 15, 32; in state department of education, 17; supervising, 9; support, 23–25, 28, 29, 30, 34, 35; types of, 22–25. *See also* Media aide; Media specialist; Media technician
Media technician, 23, 28, 29, 33–35; competencies of, 24; definition, 110; duties of, 24
Membership subscription in networks, 19–20
Microcard, 72
Microfiche, 72
Microfilm, 72
Microform equipment, 72
Microforms, school collection, 72
Microprojectors, 83
Mobile units, 16
Models, 25, 81; designing, 46
Motion pictures, *see* Films
Multi-image presentations, produced by schools, 51
Multimedia presentations, designing, 7

Networks, 19–20

Newspapers: school collection, 71; storage, 102

Offices for professional staff, 99
Opaque projectors, 82
Open access materials, facilities for, 97
Open-reel projector, 78
Overhead projectors, 74

Pamphlets, school collection, 71–72
Paper cutters, 85
Parents, informing about media program, 57
Per Pupil Operational Cost, 40–42
Periodicals: school collection, 71; storage, 102
Personnel, *see* Media staff
Photocopier, 85
Photography, 24; production, 45, 47, 91, 94; staff for, 30
Pictures, *see* Graphics
Planning media programs, 7, 11, 18, 27, 36–38
Posters, 24; school collection, 75
Presses, 84
Principal of school, 15
Print materials, school collection, 70–72
Printers: diazo, 85; microform, 72
Printing, 30; production, 45, 93; staff for, 29
Prints, school collection, 75
Problem-solving, 14
Process, 111–12; definition of, 110
Processing of materials, 24, 26, 28, 90–91
Processing services, 48, 49
Production of materials, 5, 6, 9, 11, 14, 24, 25, 29–30, 86, 91; audiotape, 86; by district, 45–46; equipment, 84–86; film, 24; graphics, 85; by school, 46–48; by students, 47–48
Professional materials in collections, 63
Professional staff, 22–23, 28, 29; definition, 109; district media director, 12, 21, 25, 26–27, 31, 38, 39, 40, 42–43, 56, 57, 87, 109–10; head of school media program, 13, 15, 21, 31–32, 38, 110; library for, 10, 14,

28, 66–67, 90, 101; offices for, 99; qualifications, 22–23; for school media program, 31–34
Projection carts, 83
Projection screens, 83–84
Projectors: cartridge-loaded, 78; filmstrip, 73; large-group equipment, 83; microprojectors, 83; opaque, 82; open-reel, 78; overhead, 74; 16mm, 77; slide, 74; stop-motion mechanism for, 77, 78; Super 8mm, 78
Public information, 9, 11, 14, 27, 32, 55–58
Purchasing, 14; guiding principles, 42–43

Qualifications for professional staff, 22–23

Radio: educational broadcast, 16, 80; production, 30, 45–46; staff for, 30; studio, 91, 102
Readers, microform, 72
Reading: area; 96; developing competencies in, 8, 15
Record players, 79
Recorders: audiotape, 79, 86; videotape, 85
Reference service, providing, 8
Region, definition of, 111
Regional media program: definition of, 111; functions of, 16; funding, 17
Remote access: distribution systems, 16; storage and control for, 102
Research programs relating to media, 18
Resources, see Materials
Retrieval systems, 20, 48
Rotary laminator, 84

School district, see District
School media center, 93–103; definition of, 111; operating, 14
School media program, 68–86; access and delivery systems, 52–53; activities responding to curriculum goals, 14; and curriculum design, 15; definition of, 111; evaluation, 15, 60–61; facilities, 92–103; head of, 13,

15, 21, 31–32, 38, 110; planning, 13, 31; production of materials, 46–48, 50–51; public information program, 32, 58; purposes of, 13, 14; responsibilities of, 13–15; scheduling, 52–53; staff for, 30–35; value for students, 15
School principal, 15
Schools: collections, 62–63, 68–86; definition of, 111; design, 93; enrollment, 92; instructional programs, 92–93; new, media programs for, 34–35; sharing of materials between, 63–64
Screens, projection, 83–84
Sculpture, 81
Self-instruction, developing materials for, 7
Skills, developing, 8, 15, 105
Slides: equipment, 74; school collection, 73–74
Small group listening and viewing, 97–98
Space, locating, 6
Specimens, 81
Stacks, facilities, 101–2
State department of education, media programs in, 17–19
State media program, 17; responsibilities, 18–19
Stop-motion mechanism for film projectors, 77, 78
Study habits, developing, 8
Super 8mm camera, 85
Supplies, purchasing, 43–44
Support staff, 23–25; for district media program, 28–30; for school media program, 35
System components, installing, 24

Tables for media center, 97
Tactile materials, 80–81
Tape recorders, 79, 85, 86
Tape splicers, 86
Teachers: informing about media program, 57; involving in school media program, 14, 60; professional resources for, 14; staff development programs for, 14, 16, 32
Technicians, see Media technicians
Technology: communication, 10; instructional, 112

Telecommunications, 10, 11, 19–20
Television, 17; closed-circuit, 84; educational, 16; office, 103; production, 30, 45–46, 91, 94; reception, 76; staff for, 30; storage, 103; studio, 103
Terminology, 109–13
Textbooks, 81–82
Thermal transparency maker, 85
Toys, 80–81
Transparencies, 24, 25, 73, 74
Transparency makers, 85
Typewriters for graphic production, 85

Users: activities in media program, 5–6, 60–61, 105, 106–107; assessment of needs and interests, 37–38, 68, 69; assisting, 8; characteristics of, 92; definition, 5; developing competencies in, 8, 15; developing understanding of media in, 8; informing about media program, 57; proportion of staff to number, 33–35

Video playback equipment, 77
Videotapes, 66, 76, 90; collections, 28; production, 46, 47
Viewers: filmstrip, 73; slide, 74
Viewing, 97–98; area for, 96–98; developing competencies in, 8
Visual materials, school collection, 73–78

Work space, facilities for, 99

6882